PocketRadiologist®
ER-Trauma
Top 100 Diagnoses

PocketRadiologist®
ER-Trauma
Top 100 Diagnoses

Robert A Novelline MD
Professor of Radiology, Harvard Medical School
Director of Emergency Radiology
Massachusetts General Hospital
Boston, MA

James T Rhea MD
Associate Professor of Radiology, Harvard Medical School
Emergency Radiologist
Harvard Medical School
Boston, MA

Thomas Ptak MD PhD MPH
Assistant Professor of Radiology, Harvard Medical School
Emergency Radiologist
Massachusetts General Hospital
Boston, MA

Faranak Sadri-Tafazoli MD
Clinical Fellow, Divison Emergency Radiology
Massachusetts General Hospital
Harvard Medical School
Boston, MA

Andrew B Small MD
Clinical Fellow, Divison Emergency Radiology
Massachusetts General Hospital
Harvard Medical School
Boston, MA

With 200 drawings and radiographic images

Drawings: Richard Coombs MS, Lane R. Bennion MS

*Image Editing: Melissa A. Morris, Cassie L. Dearth,
                  Angie D. Mascarenaz*

AMIRSYS®

W. B. SAUNDERS COMPANY
An Elsevier Science Company

AMIRSYS®

A medical reference publishing company

First Edition

First Printing: June 2004

Composition by Amirsys Inc, Salt Lake City, Utah

Printed by K/P Corp, Salt Lake City, Utah

ISBN: 0-7216-0459-5

Preface

The **PocketRadiologist**® series is an innovative, quick reference designed to deliver succinct, up-to-date information to practicing professionals "at the point of service." As close as your pocket, world-renowned authors write each title in the series. These experts have designated the "top 100" diagnoses or interventional procedures in every major body area, bulleted the most essential facts, and offered high-resolution imaging to illustrate each topic. Selected references are included for further review. Full color anatomic-pathologic computer graphics model many of the actual diseases.

Each **PocketRadiologist**® title follows an identical format. The same information is in the same place - every time - and takes you quickly from key facts to imaging findings, differential diagnosis, pathology, pathophysiology, and relevant clinical information. The interventional modules give you the essentials and "how-tos" of important procedures, including pre- and post-procedure checklists, common problems and complications.

PocketRadiologist® titles are available in both print and hand-held PDA formats. Currently available modules feature Brain, Head and Neck, Orthopaedic (Musculoskeletal) Imaging, Pediatrics, Spine, Chest, Cardiac, Vascular, Abdominal Imaging and Interventional Radiology. 2003 topics that will round out the PocketRadiologist™ series include Obstetrics, Gynecologic Imaging, Breast, Temporal Bone, Pediatric Neuroradiology and Emergency Imaging.

Anne G Osborn MD
Executive Vice President
Editor-in-Chief, Amirsys Inc

H Ric Harnsberger MD
Chairman and CEO, Amirsys Inc

Notice and Disclaimer

PocketRadiologist®
ER-Trauma
Top 100 Diagnoses

The diagnoses in this book are divided into 9 sections in the following order:

Head Injury
Face Injury
Cervical Spine/Neck Injury
Thoracic Injury
Abdominal Injury
Thoracolumbar Spine Trauma
Upper Extremity Injury
Pelvic Fractures
Lower Extremity Injury

Table of Contents

Thoracic Injury

Table of Contents

Abdominal Injury

Table of Contents

PocketRadiologist[®]

ER-Trauma

Top 100 Diagnoses

HEAD INJURY

Skull Fracture

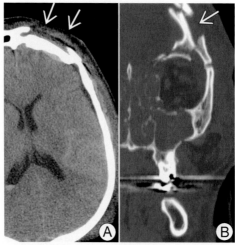

Axial CT shows depressed left frontal skull fracture (A, arrows). Note small epidural hematoma and subarachnoid hemorrhage in the left Sylvian fissure and right lateral ventricle atrium. Fracture shown on coronal reformation (B, arrow) demonstrates a depressed fragment and extension to the orbital roof.

Key Facts
- Head trauma is a major factor in death/disability in multiple trauma patients
- Skull films are not enough if trauma mechanism is sufficient for injury
- 1/3 of patients with severe brain injury don't have fracture
- Fractures can be linear, depressed, diastatic
- Skull base fractures can damage blood vessels, dura, and cranial nerves
- Sequelae include pneumocephalus, CSF leak, nerve palsy, stroke

Imaging Findings
General Features
- Linear fracture
  - Sharply delineated lucent line; does not branch
  - Overlying soft tissue swelling almost always present
- Depressed fracture
  - Fragment(s) displaced inwards
- Diastatic fracture
  - Sutures spread; may have co-existing linear fracture
  - Cranial "burst fracture"
    - Unique in infants; diastases widened > 4mm
    - Brain herniates through fracture; extrudes under scalp
- Skull base (temporal bone) fracture – longitudinal or transverse
  - Longitudinal accompanied by conductive hearing loss
    - Ossicular diastasis or tear of tympanic membrane
  - Transverse accompanied by sensory-neural hearing loss
    - Injury to cochlea or 7th/8th nerve complex
Imaging Recommendations
- Non-enhanced CT (NECT) if patient has sufficient trauma mechanism and clinical findings

Skull Fracture

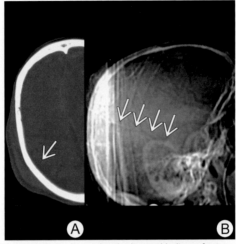

Axial NECT bone windows show a barely discernable linear fracture of the right parietal bone (A, arrow). Note overlying sub-galeal hematoma. Lateral scout view shows a linear lucency nearly parallel to the plane of the axial acquisition (B, arrows).

- o Glasgow coma scale (GCS) < 14; loss of consciousness > 30 seconds at scene
- Axial images may miss linear fractures in the plane of the image
  - o Check skull on CT scout image for obvious linear fractures
    - ▪ 10% of patients with GCS = 15 + loss of consciousness or amnesia have abnormalities on CT scan
    - ▪ 5% of patients with GCS = 15 + normal neurological exam have significant intracranial injury revealed on CT
- Use both bone, soft tissue algorithms
- View/film using 3 window settings
  - o Soft tissue (level = 40H, window-75-100H)
  - o Bone (level = 500H, window = 3,000H)
  - o Intermediate (level = 75H, window = 150-200H) for small subdural hematomas (SDHs)
    - ▪ May have to lower window in anemic patients
- Evaluate for vascular injury if carotid canal involved

Differential Diagnosis

Suture Line
- Acute fracture is lucent and has sharp, non-corticated margins
- Suture less distinct, has dense sclerotic borders

Vascular Groove
- Typical location (i.e., middle meningeal artery (MMA)), corticated margins, branching

Venous Lake
- Typical location (i.e., parasagittal), corticated margins

Arachnoid Granulation
- Typical location (parasagittal, transverse sinus), corticated margins

Skull Fracture

Pathology
<u>General</u>
- Etiology-Pathogenesis
  - Direct blunt impact to skull
    - Fracture may occur at point of direct impact or along plane of force deposition at skull base - e.g., petrous temporal bone
- Epidemiology
  - Fracture present in majority of severe head injury cases
  - 25-35% of severely injured patients do not have skull fracture
  - Skull fracture absent in 25% of fatal injuries at autopsy!

<u>Gross Pathologic or Surgical Features</u>
- Types: Linear, depressed, diastatic
- Associated injuries
  - Linear fracture: Extra-axial hematoma
    - Fracture with tear of middle meningeal artery => epidural hematoma (EDH)
    - Posterior fossa fracture + tear of dural sinus => venous EDH (rare)
  - Depressed fracture: Lacerated dura, arachnoid; parenchymal injury
  - Skull base fracture: Cranial nerve injury, CSF leak, epistaxis, periorbital bruising
  - 10-15% of patients with severe head trauma (GCS 3-6) have C1 or C2 fracture

Clinical Issues
<u>Presentation</u>
- Significant findings on presentation or at scene
  - Initial GCS < 14
  - Loss of consciousness or > 30 sec at scene
  - No recall for the incident or amnesia
  - "Star" crack of windshield

<u>Natural History</u>
- Varies with underlying injury
- Patients who return to ED have a remarkable incidence of missed intracranial lesions, poor outcome

Selected References
1. Hofman PAM et al: Value of radiological diagnosis of skull fracture in the management of mild head injury. J Neurol Neurosurg Psychiatr 68: 416-22, 2000
2. Procaccio F, et al: Guidelines for the treatment of adults with severe head trauma (part I). Initial assessment; evaluation and pre-hospital treatment; current criteria for hospital admission; systemic and cerebral monitoring. J Neurosurg Sci. 44(1):1-10, 2000
3. Vilks GM et al: Use of a complete neurological examination to screen for significant intracranial abnormalities in minor head injury. Am J Emerg Med 18: 159-63, 2000

Subdural Hematoma (SDH)

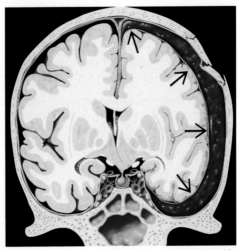

Coronal drawing shows subdural collection with the membrane bound brain (arrows) pushed away from the inner table of the skull, giving the classic "crescent" appearance.

Key Facts
- Density decreases approximately 1.5H/day as SDH evolves
- > 70% of acute SDHs have significant associated lesions
- Use low level (30-50H) and wide window settings (150-200H)

Imaging Findings
<u>General Features</u>
- Diagnostic clue = compressed sulci uniform, displaced inward from skull
- Acute (aSDH) and subacute (sSDH)
  - Crescentic collection over hemisphere
  - May cross sutures, not dural attachments
  - Often extends into interhemispheric fissure, along tentorium
  - Other lesions (e.g., traumatic SAH) in > 70%
- Chronic SDH (cSDH)
  - Crescentic, or may be low (fluid) density lentiform mass
  - Fluid hematoma + encapsulating membranes
  - Recurrent, mixed-age post traumatic SDH common
    - **In children with mixed cSDH, consider nonaccidental trauma!**

<u>CT Findings</u>
- aSDH (immediate to several days)
  - 60% high density (clot organizes in first 1-2 hours after bleed)
  - 40% mixed hyper-, hypodense (active bleed or torn arachnoid)
  - Hyperacute (unclotted) aSDH mostly hypodense
  - May be isodense if coagulopathy/anemia (Hgb < 8-10g/dl)
- sSDH (2 days-2 weeks after formation)
  - May be same density as underlying cortex
  - Gray-white junction displaced medially
  - CSF in compressed sulci under SDH
  - IV contrast may enhance displaced cortical veins

Subdural Hematoma (SDH)

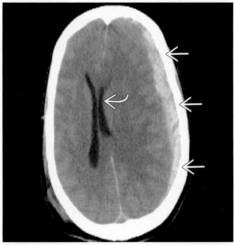

Acute SDH showing classic hyperdense "crescent" shape. Sulci are compressed and cortical boundary appears uniform and pushed centrally away from the inner table of the skull (arrows). Ventricles are effaced with movement of mass across midline through the falcine hiatus "subfalcine herniation" seen (curved arrow).

- cSDH (weeks-months after formation) can be classified by internal architecture/extension
  - Homogeneous
    - Homogeneous density
    - Can be laminar (thin, high density layer of fresh blood along inner membrane)
  - Separated
    - Layered components (high density bottom, low density top)
    - Density may gradually change from low to high from the anti-dependent to dependent position of the hematoma ("graded")
  - Trabeculated
    - Heterogeneous with high density septa
    - Contents low to isodense
    - Thickened or calcified capsule
  - Other findings of cSDH
    - IV contrast shows neovascularity in organizing membranes
    - +/- "Hygroma" (subdural CSF, arachnoid tear)
    - 1-2% calcify

MR Findings
- Signal varies with hematoma age
- cSDH
  - Membranes enhance
  - Leaky neovascularity
  - Delayed scans show contrast diffuse into SDH

Differential Diagnosis
cSDH
- Subdural hygroma (clear CSF, no encapsulating membranes)
- Subdural effusion (xanthochromic fluid from extravasation of plasma from outer membrane; 20% evolve into cSDH)

Subdural Hematoma (SDH)

- Pachymeningopathies (thickened dura)
  - Chronic meningitis (may be indistinguishable)
  - Post-surgical (shunt, etc.)
  - Intracranial hypotension ("slumping" midbrain, tonsillar herniation)
  - Sarcoid (nodular, "lumpy-bumpy")
  - Metastases (skull often involved)

Pathology
General
- Etiology-Pathogenesis
  - aSDH
    - Occur by both inertial and direct impact injury
    - Sudden tangential linear or angular acceleration
    - Parasagittal bridging veins disrupted
    - Blood collects between dural layer and arachnoid membrane
    - Thrombin forms clot by crosslinking and organizing
    - Increases in density from ~ 35-45H to ~ 60-80H
  - sSDH
    - Clot and RBCs begin lysis and resorption, Hgb degrades
    - Density decreases an average of 1.5H/day
  - cSDH
    - Develops over 2-3 weeks
    - Serosanguineous fluid with heme byproducts
    - Encapsulated by granulation tissue
    - "Neomembranes" with fragile capillaries
    - Cycle of recurrent bleeding-coagulation-fibrinolysis
    - 5% multiloculated with fluid-blood density levels
    - May continue to enlarge
- Epidemiology
  - SDHs found in 10-20% of imaged, 30% of autopsy cases

Clinical Issues
Presentation
- Loss of consciousness, seizure, focal deficits due to brain compression, venous congestion and eventually herniation
Treatment & Prognosis
- Prognosis in aSDH poor (50% mortality)
  - IV Mannitol within the first 6 hours of injury may improve outcome
- Hematoma thickness, midline shift > 20 mm correlate with poor outcome
- Lethal if hematoma volume > 8-10% of intracranial volume
- Recurrence risk of cSDH varies with type ("separated" is highest; fragile neovessels disappear in thickened or calcified neomembrane, therefore very low likelihood of re-hemorrhages)

Selected References
1. Lee KS: Review of the Natural Evolution of Subdural Hematomas. Brain Inj (18)4:351-8, 2004
2. Nakaguchi H et al: Factors in the natural history of chronic subdural hematomas that influence their postoperative recurrence. J Neurosug 95:256-62, 2001
3. Kaminogo M et al: Characteristics of symptomatic chronic subdural haematomas on high-field MRI. Neuroradiol 41:109-16, 1999

Epidural Hematoma (EDH)

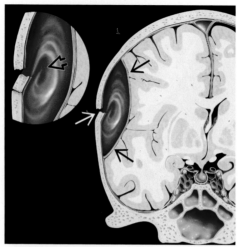

Coronal drawing shows a depressed skull fracture (white arrow), with epidural hematoma (black arrows indicate displaced dura). Magnified view shows transected artery in red with "swirl" (open arrow) indicating active bleeding.

Key Facts
- Uncommon, potentially fatal
- Prompt recognition, appropriate treatment essential
- Classic "lucid interval" in < 50%
- Hypoattenuating area ("swirl sign") = acute bleeding
- 10-25% show delayed enlargement

Imaging Findings
General Features
- Best diagnostic sign = hyperdense biconvex extra-axial mass
- Underlying brain, subarachnoid space compressed
- Gray-white interface displaced
- Herniation common

CT Findings
- Skull fracture in 85-90%
- Nearly all EDHs occur at impact ("coup") site
- 2/3 hyperdense; 1/3 mixed hyper/hypo
  - Low density "swirl sign" = active bleeding
  - Gas bubbles up to 20%
- 1/3-1/2 have other significant lesions
  - "Contrecoup" SDH
  - Contusions
- Secondary effects common
  - Perfusion alterations
  - Herniations (subfalcine, descending transtentorial)

MR Findings
- Thin black line between EDH, brain = displaced dura
- Acute EDH isointense with cortex on most sequences

Other Modality Findings
- DSA

Epidural Hematoma (EDH)

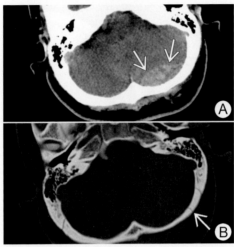

(A) NECT scan shows mildly heterogeneous epidural hematoma in the posterior fossa (arrows). (B) Bone windows show a skull fracture that crosses the left transverse sinus (arrow). This epidural hematoma originated as a result of venous hemorrhage into the epidural space.

- o Avascular lentiform-shaped mass
- o Cortical arteries displaced away from skull
- o May displace dural venous sinus
- o Middle meningeal artery (MMA) laceration (rare)
  - ▪ "Tram track" sign (contrast extravasates from MMA into paired middle meningeal veins)
- MRA
  - o Demonstrates displaced venous sinus, if present

Differential Diagnosis
<u>Nontraumatic Hyperdense Extra-Axial Masses</u>
- Meningioma (enhances)
- Metastasis (adjacent skull lesion common)
- Dural tuberculoma (enhances)
- Extramedullary hematopoiesis (history of blood dyscrasia)

Pathology
<u>General</u>
- Etiology-Pathogenesis (lacerated vessel)
  - o 85-90% MMA
  - o 10-15% other (dural sinus)
- Epidemiology
  - o 1-4% of imaged trauma patients
  - o 10% autopsy prevalence
<u>Gross Pathologic, Surgical Features</u>
- Hematoma collects between calvarium, outer dura
  - o Temporoparietal most common site
  - o May cross midline, dural attachments
  - o Rarely crosses sutures (exception: Large hematoma, diastatic fracture)

Epidural Hematoma (EDH)

- > 95% unilateral
- 90-95% supratentorial
- Uncommon
  - 5-10% posterior fossa
  - "Vertex" EDH
    - Rare
    - Linear or diastatic fracture crosses (superior sagittal sinus (SSS))
    - Usually venous
    - Size underestimated on axial CT

Clinical Issues

Presentation

- Classic "lucid interval" in < 50%
- Signs of mass effect, herniation common
- Pupil-involving CN III palsy

Natural History

- Delayed development or enlargement common
  - 10-25% of cases
  - Usually occurs within first 36 hours

Treatment & Prognosis

- Generally good outcome if promptly recognized, treated
  - 5% overall mortality
- Even large volume EDHs can have low morbidity
- Small EDHs sometimes followed without surgery

Selected references
1. Al-Nakshabandi NA: The swirl sign. Radiol 218:433, 2001
2. Sullivan TP et al: Follow-up of conservatively managed epidural hematomas. AJNR 20: 107-13, 1999
3. Paterniti S et al: Is the size of an epidural hematoma related to outcome? Acta Neurochir 140:953-5, 1998

Traumatic Subarachnoid (tSAH)

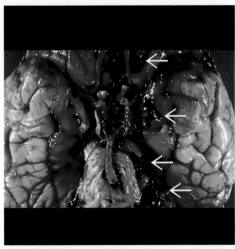

Autopsy specimen shows clotted blood layering the under surface of the brain in the ambient, pre-pontine and supra-sellar cisterns and the sub-frontal subarachnoid space (arrows). Sulci are swollen with flattened crests from diffuse brain swelling.

Key Facts
- Trauma is most common cause of SAH (**not** ruptured aneurysm!)
- Amount of tSAH correlates with complications leading to delayed ischemia and poor outcome

Imaging Findings
General Features
- Best diagnostic sign = high density in gravity dependent sulci and in basal cisterns
- Looks identical to aneurysmal SAH (aSAH) except for location
  - Adjacent to other injuries along plane of force (coup, contre-coup)
  - Note: Subarachnoid blood is displaced with CSF pulsations
  - Though it is usually in these places, it can be anywhere in the CSF space
  - Check convexity sulci, dependent portion of sylvian-fissure, basal cisterns
CT Findings
- tSAH
  - High density in subarachnoid space(s)
  - Blood in interpeduncular cistern or "notch" (gravity dependent)
    - May be only manifestation of subtle SAH
- Traumatic intraventricular hemorrhage (tIVH)
  - High density in dependent portion of ventricles i.e., lateral recesses of 4th, posterior 3rd, atria of lateral
  - Blood-CSF level common
MR Findings
- Note: Blood signal changes with time and MR sequence
  - Hyperacute blood separates (hematocrit sign) giving water signal on top and cell signal (T1 Iso, T2 Hypo) in lower layer
  - Acute tSAH (< 1hr) - clot has become a cross linked uniform gel

Traumatic Subarachnoid (tSAH)

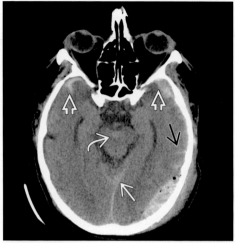

NECT scan shows that hyperdense hemorrhage falls dependently into, and takes on the shape of the inter-peduncular cistern (curved arrow), tectal plate/superior cerebellar cistern (white arrow) left temporal sulci (black arrow) and bilateral anterior temporal pole sulci (open arrows).

- Isointense to brain on T1WI ("dirty" CSF), iso to hypointense on T2WI and hyperintense on FLAIR

Differential Diagnosis
Aneurysmal SAH
- Aneurysm can be identified on DSA/CTA/MRA in > 85%
- Contusions, SDH, other lesions present in nearly all cases of tSAH

Pathology
General
- Etiology-Pathogenesis
  - tSAH usually associated with contusions, SDH; probably arises from tearing of veins in subarachnoid space or leakage from contused cortex
  - tIVH probably arises from shearing of choroid glomus or vessels
  - Blood usually found where it formed, but blood products can be propelled by CSF pulsations or settle into gravity dependent positions – don't only look near expected site of impact
- Epidemiology
  - tSAH
    - More common than both SDH and EDH
    - Occurs in up to 45% of post trauma cases
    - 33% of SAH cases will have moderate brain injury
    - CT 95% sensitive with high specificity
    - tSAH-associated vasospasm occurs less frequently than in aneurysm associated SAH
  - tIVH
    - Uncommon, Isolated tIVH occurs in 5% of cases
    - Reflects severity of overall trauma

Traumatic Subarachnoid (tSAH)

- • Usually occurs with other injuries (i.e., deep hematomas)
- • Risk of obstructive hydrocephalus

<u>Gross Pathologic, Surgical Features</u>
- • tSAH: Acute blood in convexity sulci, fissures and cisterns
- • tIVH: Blood-CSF levels in ventricles

Clinical Issues
<u>Presentation</u>
- • Depends on associated injuries

<u>Natural History</u>
- • tSAH
  - o Acute hydrocephalus rare
  - o Vasospasm
    - • May develop quickly (2-3 days post-injury)
    - • Peaks 2 weeks after injury
    - • Uncommon cause of post traumatic infarct
- • tIVH
  - o Rarely may develop intra- or extra-ventricular obstructive hydrocephalus

<u>Treatment & Prognosis</u>
- • tSAH
  - o Degree of tSAH on initial CT scan correlates with poor outcome
- • tIVH
  - o Gradually clears

Selected References
1. Server A et al: Post-traumatic cerebral infarction. Acta Radiol 42: 254-60, 2001
2. Gentry LR: Imaging of closed head injury. Radiol 191: 1-17, 1994
3. Fisher CM et al: Relation of cerebral vasospasm to subarachnoid hemorrhage visualized by computerized tomographic scanning. Neurosurgery Jan 6(1):1-9, 1980

Cerebral Contusion

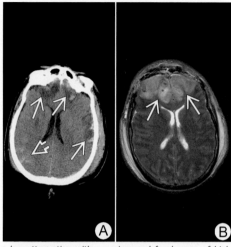

NECT shows low attenuation with superimposed focal areas of high attenuation representing hemorrhagic contusion in the frontal and left temporal lobes (A, arrows). Subarachnoid blood has no surrounding edema (A, open arrow). Axial T2WI MR scan shows bilateral swollen, hyper intense frontal lobes (B, arrows).

Key Facts
- Synonyms: Contusion, brain bruise, hemorrhagic contusion
- Direct impact injury to the brain parenchyma
- Typically occurs in the cortical mantle and superficial white matter, but can occur in deep white matter with sufficient impact
  - Direct impact of brain with inner table of skull or fibrous skull compartment ligament (e.g., falx, tentorium, petro-clival ligament)
- Occurs commonly in typical locations
  - Frontal pole and sub frontal mantle, anterior temporal pole, fronto-parietal convexity

Imaging Findings
General Features
- Best imaging clue: Low attenuation cortical mantle and white matter infundibulum edema
- Other features: Early after injury, edema may not be evident; may see
  - Swollen or expanded gyri/focally effaced sulci
  - Parenchymal hemorrhage, especially peripheral
- Anatomy: Injury most prominent at point of impact: Gyri rectus, medial, anterior and posterior orbital gyri, superior and middle temporal gyri and posterior frontal convexity/para central lobule region
- Can extend deep if severe impact
- Deep white matter injuries (beyond the gray-white junction) tend to favor diffuse axonal injury
CT Findings
- NECT shows expanded gyri or sulcal effacement

Cerebral Contusion

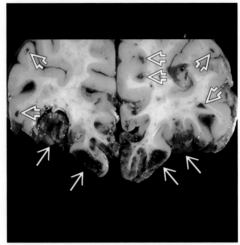

Coronal cut section of autopsy specimen shows coarse, dark micro hemorrhage following the gyral crests of the bilateral gyri rectus, medial and lateral orbital gyri (arrows). Red punctate lesions situated in the gray-white junction and left inferior frontal white matter (open arrows) represent diffuse axonal injury.

- Gray matter is iso- to hypodense with low attenuation extending into peripheral white matter
- Most subtle cases, swollen gyri with loss of gray-white differentiation
- CECT shows above architecture, but may show pial enhancement due to loss of blood-brain barrier or destruction of capillaries
- Cortex may be hypoperfused due to congestion and local swelling

MR Findings
- T1WI: Swollen gyri are iso- to hypo intense with respect to normal signal
- Low signal extends into local white matter infundibular
- T2WI: Swollen gyri are hyper intense with respect to normal signal
- Hyperintensity extends into local white matter
- Gray and white matter differentiation is lost
- Gradient echo susceptibility sequences may show iso- to markedly hypo intense foci representing punctate hemorrhage with greater sensitivity

Imaging Recommendations
- NECT is currently best first line imaging to assess parenchymal injury as well as extra and intra axial hemorrhage
- MRI is second line, mostly due to access and length of imaging time in severely injured patients, but is most sensitive for parenchymal injury

Differential Diagnosis

Laceration
- Represents an extreme of force deposition
- Instead of causing micro traumatic injury to neuropil and microvasculature, gross tear of the parenchyma with hemorrhage

Subarachnoid Hemorrhage
- Iso- to hyperdense hemorrhage layering in sulci may give the appearance of swollen gyri or cortical hemorrhage

Cerebral Contusion

Pathology

General

- General Path Comments
  - Injury is typically in the most cranial surfaces of the neuraxis (e.g., sub frontal surface, frontal poles, temporal poles frontal convexity) and surfaces adjacent to fixed tendon compartmental dividers (e.g., tentorium, falx)
- Etiology-Pathogenesis
  - Direct impact causes tissue compressive forces on superficial cortical layers
  - Crush injury to neuropil on compression with tensile force injury on elastic recoil
  - Tensile and shear forces within neuropil tear capillaries and arterioles

Gross Pathologic, Surgical Features

- Injured gray matter ribbon is friable and shows course granular texture with dark reddish-brown color instead of smooth grayish-pink appearance

Microscopic Features

- Groups of punctate hemorrhages at right angle to cortex
- Blood extends along the vessels to the adjacent cortex where local neurons undergo necrosis
- Later there is proliferation of capillaries, astrocytes and microglia
- Dead tissue is removed, replaced by shrunken, gliotic fenestrated scar containing residual hemosiderin filled macrophages

Clinical Issues

Presentation

- Ranges from mild concussion (confusion, disorientation, cognitive decline, headache) to seizures, motor or sensory disturbance and coma depending on the degree and volume of injured tissue

Natural History

- Impact/injury, micro injury to neuropil and capillaries; micro hemorrhage, disturbance of cerebral auto regulation, edema/swelling, volume, mass effect, cortical ischemia/congestion, ischemic injury, additional swelling/edema, herniation syndromes, if survive above encephalomalacia, gliosis, seizures, neural deficit

Treatment & Prognosis

- Control intra cranial pressure (osmotic diuresis, steroids, hyperventilation)
- Seizure control
- Depends on volume and extent of injury and function affected
- In one series, 16.8% of patients with GCS 3-8; 24.3% with GCS 9-12; and 8% with GCS 13-15 developed seizures over 24 month follow-up

Selected References
1. Hardman JM et al: Pathology of head trauma. J Neuroimaging Clin N Am May;12(2):175-87, 2002
2. Marik PE et al: Management of head trauma. Chest. Aug;122(2):699-711, 2002
3. Zee CS et al: Imaging of head trauma. Neuroimaging Clin N Am. May;12(2):325-38, 2002

Diffuse Axonal Injury

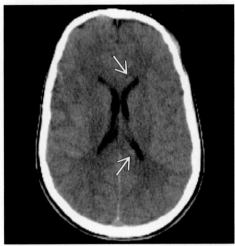

NECT in a multiple trauma patient with GCS = 6 shows subtle hyperdensities in the left corpus callosum genu and periatrial splenium (arrows).

Key Facts
- Diffuse axonal injury (DAI) = second most common traumatic brain injury (TBI)
- Axons **not** mechanically "sheared", but stretched (tensile stress)
- Impaired axoplasmic transport, axonal swelling, disconnection
- Most DAI lesions are microscopic, nonhemorrhagic
- MR is superior to CT for detection

Imaging Findings
General Features
- Multiple lesions in nearly all cases
- Best diagnostic sign = hemorrhages at gray/white matter, corpus callosum, fornix, upper brainstem, basal ganglia, internal capsule
CT Findings
- May be normal, especially with mild TBI
- 20-50% demonstrate petechial hemorrhage(s)
- 10-20% evolve to focal mass lesion
MR Findings
- Multiple high signal foci on T2WI, FLAIR
- Low signal on T2* ("susceptibility weighted") sequences
Other Modality Findings
- Decreased ADC
- Magnetic resonance spectroscopic (MRS): Decreased NAA/Cr correlates with outcome
- Medium scale integration (MSI): Abnormal low-frequency magnetic activity
Imaging Recommendations
- Follow-up at 24h (1/6 evolve)

Diffuse Axonal Injury

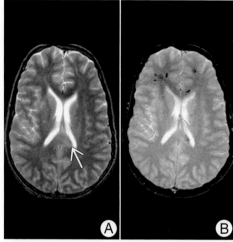

T2WI in same multiple trauma patient as shown on previous page shows hyper intensity in left posterior corpus callosum (A, arrow), but other foci are not evident. Gradient echo MRI (B) demonstrates more extensive "blooming" hypo intensities, indicating more sites of axonal injury than expected from NECT or T2W MRI.

Differential Diagnosis
Nonhemorrhagic DAI
- Multifocal white matter hyperintensities on T2WI
  - Demyelinating disease (ovoid, may enhance)
  - Small vessel disease, lacunar infarcts (older patients)
  - Metastases (enhance)

Hemorrhagic DAI
- Multiple "black dots" on T2W and T2*
  - Hypertensive microhemorrhages (longstanding chronic HTN)
  - Amyloid angiopathy (elderly, normotensive, often demented)
  - Cavernous/capillary malformations (mixed hemorrhages)

Pathology
General
- Etiology-Pathogenesis
  - Inertial forces in nonimpact injuries
  - Rapid head rotation
  - Differential acceleration/deceleration
  - Axons rarely disconnected or "sheared" (only in most severe injury)
  - Non-disruptively injured axons undergo
    - Traumatic depolarization
    - Massive ion fluxes, spreading depression
    - Excitatory amino acid release
    - Metabolic alterations
    - Cellular swelling
    - Accelerated glycolysis, lactate accumulation
  - Result
    - Secondary "axotomy"
    - Impaired axoplasmic transport

- ▪ Disconnection
- ▪ Wallerian degeneration, diffuse de-afferentation
- Epidemiology
  - o Second most common lesion in traumatic brain injury
  - o Occurs in slightly less than 50% of cases
  - o 80-100% autopsy prevalence in fatal injuries

Gross Pathologic, Surgical Features
- Multiple small round/ovoid/linear white matter lesions
- Widely distributed
  - o Parasagittal white matter
  - o Corpus callosum
  - o Brain stem tracts (e.g., medial lemnisci, corticospinal tracts)

Microscopic Features
- Axonal swellings, "retraction" balls
- Microglial clusters
- Macro-, microhemorrhages (torn penetrating vessels)

Clinical Issues

Presentation
- Immediate coma typical
- Brainstem damage (pontomedullary rent) associated with immediate or early death
- Mild DAI can occur without coma

Natural History
- Variable course
- Post-concussion syndrome (persistent headache, cognitive decline, personality changes)

Treatment & Prognosis
- Variable: TBI = 80% mild, 10% moderate, 10% severe
- Admission GCS does not always correlate with outcome
- In absence of expanding mass lesion (e.g., EDH) DAI is most common cause of post-traumatic coma, vegetative state
- Significant genomic responses to brain trauma occur
  - o Induction of "immediate early genes"
  - o Activation of multiple signal transduction pathways
  - o Apolipoprotein E (apoE) genotype, amyloid deposition may influence clinical outcome

Selected References
1. Sinson G et al: MTI and proton MRS in the evaluation of axonal injury. AJNR 22:143-51, 2001
2. Kuzma BB et al: Improved identification of axonal shear injuries with gradient echo MR technique. Surg Neurol 53:400-2, 2000
3. Graham DI et al: Neurotrauma. Brain Pathol 7:1285-8, 1997

Cerebral Herniation

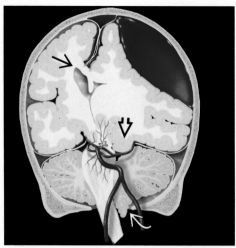

Coronal drawing shows rightward subfalcine herniation (arrow), left transtentorial herniation (open arrow) and left tonsillar herniation (curved arrow).

Key Facts
- Secondary effects include herniation, increased ICP, altered blood flow and fluid re-distribution (3rd spacing) worsen the severity of initial injury
- Secondary effects are often more devastating than primary injury

Imaging Findings
General Features
- Best diagnostic sign = displaced or effaced ventricles and cisterns
- Brain, vessels shifted from one compartment into another

CT Findings
- Subfalcine herniation
  - Septum pellucidum not at midline
  - Cingulate gyrus displaced under falx
  - Lateral ventricles and corpus callosum displaced away from lesion
  - Ipsilateral ventricle compressed
  - Foramen of Monro obstructs - contralateral lateral ventricle enlarges (= trapped ventricle)
  - Anterior cerebral artery (ACA) displaced across midline
    - May become pinned against falx and occluded
    - May cause frontal infarct - late
- Unilateral descending transtentorial (uncal) herniation
  - Early
    - Uncus, parahippocampal gyrus migrate medially
    - Ipsilateral suprasellar (ambient and sylvian) cistern effaced
    - Ipsilateral CN III compressed
    - Pons leans or twists as it is pushed downward
    - Asymmetric widening of ipsilateral ambient cistern
  - Late
    - Suprasellar cistern completely obliterated
    - Brainstem shifts away from mass
    - Becomes compressed against tent = "Kernohan notch"

Cerebral Herniation

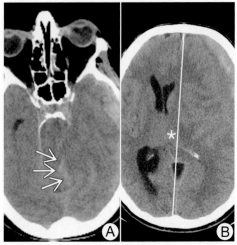

(A) NECT shows transtentorial herniation with obliteration of perimesencephalic and suprasellar cisterns by soft tissue. Left temporal lobe herniates across tent edge and down (arrows). (B) Subfalcine herniation with displacement of the septum pellucidum and deep nuclei across midline (left thalamus at asterisk).

- Posterior cerebral artery (PCA) displaced inferomedially, may occlude over tent
- May result in occipital infarct
- Bilateral descending transtentorial (central) herniation
  o Severe uni- or bilateral supratentorial mass effect
  o Both hemispheres, basal nuclei pushed downwards
  o Diencephalon, midbrain displaced inferiorly through incisura
  o Both temporal lobes herniate into tentorial hiatus
  o Penetrating arteries often occlude, cause basal infarcts
- Ascending transtentorial herniation
  o Vermis, cerebellum pushed up through incisura
  o Quadrigeminal plate cistern deformed and midbrain pushed anteriorly - may obstruct aqueduct causing hydrocephalus
- Tonsillar herniation
  o Tonsils pushed down, impacted into foramen magnum
  o Cisterna magna obliterated
  o Fourth ventricle may obstruct – cause obstructive hydrocephalus

MR Findings
- Descending transtentorial herniation
  o Findings on axial and coronal studies similar to CT
  o Sagittal
    - Midbrain displaced inferiorly ("slumps")
    - Angle between midbrain and pons becomes more acute
    - Optic chiasm/hypothalamus are displaced downwards, draped over sella
    - +/- Secondary tonsillar herniation
- Hemodynamic effects of herniations
  o Diffuse perfusion disturbances
  o Vascular occlusion, infarcts
  o Diffuse cerebral edema and/or gyral swelling

Cerebral Herniation

Differential Diagnosis
- None relevant to this case

Pathology
<u>General</u>
- Etiology-Pathogenesis
  - Hemorrhage, extracellular fluid accumulate within closed space
  - CSF spaces (cisterns, ventricles) initially compressed
  - If added intracranial volume can't be accommodated
    - Gross mechanical displacement of brain
    - Brain herniates
  - May cause secondary ischemia, infarction
    - PCA occlusion, occipital infarct most common
    - ACA occlusion, distal (cingulate gyrus) infarcts
    - Perforating vessels, basal ganglia, capsule infarcts
    - Midbrain ("Duret") hemorrhage

<u>Gross Pathologic or Surgical Features</u>
- Grossly swollen, edematous brain
- Gyri compressed, flattened against calvarium
- Sulci effaced

Clinical Issues
<u>Presentation</u>
- Pupil – CN III palsy – (ipsilateral to side of lesion)
- Decreased brainstem blood flow, cardiovascular collapse
- Decerebrate posturing
- Kernohan notch
  - Ipsilateral hemiplegia (compression of opposite cerebral peduncle against tentorium)

<u>Natural History</u>
- Brain death if intracranial pressure and mass affect progress

<u>Treatment Issues</u>
- Remove pressure-causing mass or collection
- Control swelling and secondary injury caused by increased pressure
- Prolonged posttraumatic brain hypersensitivity
  - May offer potential "therapeutic window"
  - Possible use of neuroprotective agents

Selected References
1. Juul N et al: Intracranial hypertension and cerebral perfusion pressure. J Neurosurg 92: 1-6, 2000
2. Laine FJ et al: Acquired intracranial herniations. AJR 165: 967-73, 1995
3. Povlishock JT et al: Are the pathobiological changes evoked by traumatic brain injury immediate and irreversible? Brain Pathol 5: 415-26, 1995

PocketRadiologist®
ER-Trauma
Top 100 Diagnoses

FACE INJURY

Orbital Blowout Fracture

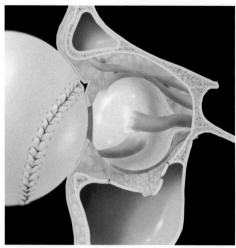

Orbital blowout fracture. Drawing illustrating mechanism for producing an orbital floor blowout fracture

Key Facts

- Synonyms: Orbital floor fracture
- Definition: Fracture of one of the walls or floor of orbit with an intact orbital rim
- Classic imaging appearance: Disruption of orbital floor with secondary findings of blood in the maxillary sinus and air in the orbit
- Other key facts
  - The most common orbital fracture
  - Produced by blow to orbit which increases intraorbital pressure, fracturing a portion of the orbital bony lining
  - May involve orbital floor, medial wall, lateral wall or orbital roof
  - Orbital floor blowout fracture most common
  - Medial wall blowout fracture second most common
  - Patients may present with pain, enophthalmos and diplopia
  - CT is optimal imaging modality

Imaging Findings

General Features

- Anatomy
  - Bones of orbital floor & medial wall are extremely thin; fracture easily
  - Orbital floor is composed of contributions from maxillary, zygomatic and palatine bones

Plain Film Findings

- Opacification of ipsilateral maxillary sinus
  - If films taken upright, see air-fluid level in maxillary sinus
- Ipsilateral orbital emphysema
- Displacement of bony fragments into maxillary sinus with floor fracture
- "Trapdoor" fragment of bone protruding downward into the sinus, often "hinged" on the ethmoidal side
- Soft tissue mass in roof of maxillary sinus representing herniated

Orbital Blowout Fracture

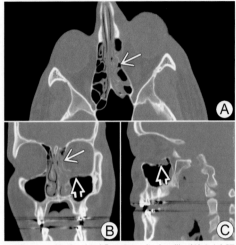

Orbital Blowout Fracture (Both orbital floor & medical wall). (A) Axial CT shows a left orbit blowout fracture (arrow) of the medial wall. (B) Coronal reformation shows the medial wall fracture (arrow) & a blowout fracture (open arrow) of orbital floor. (C) Sagittal reformation shows the left orbital floor fracture (open arrow).

- Displacement of bony fragments into ethmoid sinus with medical wall blowout fracture

CT Findings
- All findings observed on plain films with greater detail
- Any additional facial fractures and soft tissue injuries
- Associated ocular injuries
  - Lens dislocation and subluxation; corneal laceration with loss of aqueous; globe rupture; vitreous hemorrhage; subchorionic hemorrhage

Imaging Recommendations
- Plain film facial series
  - Orbital blowout fracture best seen on Water's and Caldwell views
- Face CT scan
  - Procedure of choice of imaging orbital fractures
  - 1.25 mm slices in the axial plan with coronal and sagittal reformations
  - View CT slices with both bone and soft tissue windows so not to overlook soft tissue injuries within the orbital or elsewhere

Differential Diagnosis

Zygoma Complex Fracture
- The orbital floor is fractured, but there are also fractures of the inferior orbital rim and disruption at the suture lines between the zygoma bone and the maxillary, frontal, temporal and sphenoid bones

Pathology

General
- General path comments
  - Usually orbital floor fractures but any of the orbital walls may fracture

Orbital Blowout Fracture

- o Floor and wall fractures may occur together
- o Blowout fractures increase orbital volume resulting in enophthalmos
- o Inferior rectus muscle may become entrapped with floor fractures
- o 24% of orbital blowout fractures are associated with an ocular injury
- o Blowout fractures can occur as isolated injuries on in combination with other facial fractures
  - Zygoma fractures
  - LeFort II and III fractures
  - Orbital rim fractures
- Etiology
  - o Caused by blow to eye by object that is too large to enter orbit
    - Assault, fist striking the eye; motor vehicle collision, face strikes windshield; fall onto the face
  - o Mechanism is a sudden increase in intraorbital pressure which causes fracturing of the thin bony lining of the orbit
- Epidemiology
  - o Orbital fractures are the most common facial fractures after nasal fractures
  - o Injury is more common in males in third decade

Classification
- Pure orbital blowout fracture
  - o Isolated floor or wall fracture with intact orbital rim
- Impure orbital blowout fracture
  - o Orbital rim is also fractured
- Classification also by region of orbital lining which fractures

Clinical Issues
Presentation
- Orbital pain and edema, decreased visual acuity, diplopia, numbness in distribution of infraorbital nerve, eyelid swelling when blowing nose, enophthalmos due to increase volume of bony orbit, decreased ocular motion due to entrapment of or impingement of extra-ocular muscles

Natural History
- Complications of blowout fractures include ruptured globe, persistent diplopia, neuralgia, extraocular muscle dysfunction, late/persistent enophthalmos

Treatment & Prognosis
- No treatment for minimally displaced fractures
- Surgical correction for more severe injuries with diplopia and cosmetic enophthalmos
- Good with correct diagnosis and optimal treatment
- Postoperative complications include persistent enophthalmos and diplopia

Selected References
1. Rhea JT et al: The Face. Radiology of Skeletal Trauma. Ed by Rogers LF. Churchill Livingston, Philadelphia, 3rd ed. Vol 1:315-75, 2002
2. Rhea Jt et al: Helical CT and three-dimensional CT of facial and orbital injury. Radiol Clin North Am 37:489-513, 1999
3. Novelline RA: Three dimensional computed tomography of facial trauma. Current practice in radiology. Thrall JH, ed. Mosby-Year Book, Philadelphia, PA 323-35, 1993

Nasal Fracture

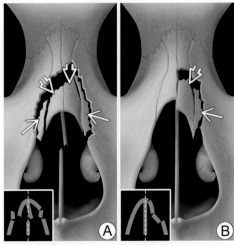

Nasal fracture mechanisms. (A) Frontal blow drawing shows posteriorly displaced fractures of both nasal bones (open arrows) and both frontal processes of maxillae (arrows). (B) Lateral blow drawing showing medially displaced fractures of the left nasal bone (open arrow) and left frontal process of maxilla (arrow).

Key Facts
- Synonym(s): Nasal trauma, nose fracture, broken nose
- Definition: Fracture of the nasal bones, frontal processes of the maxillae, and/or inferior nasal spines of the maxillae
- Other key facts
  - Most common facial fracture
    - Third most common broken bone in the body
  - The most commonly overlooked facial fracture
  - Produced by frontal or lateral blows
  - Image with plain films or CT
  - Untreated or poorly treated fractures may result in cosmetic deformity and airway obstruction

Imaging Findings
General Features
- Anatomy: Nose consists of paired nasal bones and frontal processes of the maxillae
  - Nasal bones are thick proximally at their attachment to the frontal bones and thin distally where they attach to the upper lateral cartilages
  - Nasal septum as well as the vomer and perpendicular plate of ethmoid bones separate the two airways
Plain Film Findings
- Nasal film series
  - Can show fractures of the nasal bones, frontal processes of maxillae and the inferior nasal spines of the maxillae
- Facial films series
  - Can show associated fractures in other regions of the face
  - A lateral plain film view of the face may overexpose that nasal bones such that a nasal bone fracture could be missed
    - A lateral nasal film has less exposure & better shows nasal bones

Nasal Fracture

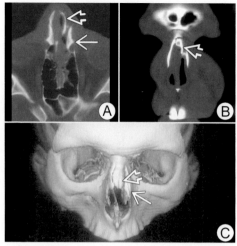

Nasal fracture (lateral blow). (A) Axial CT shows medial displacement of left nasal bone (open arrow) and posterior displacement of left frontal process of maxilla (arrow). (B) Coronal scan shows nasal bone fracture (open arrow). (C). 3D reformation shows nasal (open arrow) and frontal process (arrow) fractures.

- o Recognize the normal nasomaxillary sutures and the grooves for the nasociliary nerves
  - ▪ Do not confuse these lucencies with fractures
  - ▪ Fractures are usually perpendicular to these lucencies

CT Findings
- Best imaging modality for evaluation of suspected nasal fractures
- Will show all fractures, position and alignment of fracture fragments and associated soft tissue injuries
- Will show any associated fractures in other regions of the face

Imaging Recommendations
- Plain film exam if CT not available
  - o Nasal series: Lateral view of the nose, an occlusal view of the nose and a Water's view of the face
  - o Facial film series
    - ▪ AP, Water's, Caldwell, Towne's, base and lateral views of the face
- Face CT Scan: 1.5 mm slices of the face from above the frontal sinuses to below the mandible
  - o Routine coronal and sagittal reformations for every case

Differential Diagnosis
Naso-Orbital-Ethmoidal Fracture
- In addition to the fractures of nasal bones and frontal processes of the maxillae, there are also fractures of the medial rims of the orbits, the anterior walls of maxillary sinuses and the ethmoid sinuses
- The fracture fragments are often displaced posteriorly into the ethmoid sinuses

Nasal Fracture

Pathology

General

- General Path Comments
  - Fractures may involve the nasal bones, frontal processes of the maxillae or the inferior nasal spines of the maxillae
  - Frontal blow
    - May only be an infracture of the tips of the nasal bones or produce a severe flattening of the nasal bones and septum
    - With severe blow splaying of the nasal bones with widening of the nasal width may occur
  - Lateral blow
    - May fracture only ipsilateral nasal bone or be forceful enough to fracture the contralateral nasal bone
    - The septum may be fractured and dislocated
- Etiology-Pathogenesis
  - Usually from blunt trauma
  - Frontal blows
    - Motor vehicle collisions; patients face strikes windshield or dashboard
    - Falls onto the face
  - Lateral blows: Assaults; sports-related injuries
- Epidemiology
  - Most common facial fracture

Clinical Issues

Presentation

- Pain, edema, periorbital ecchymosis, nasal congestion, epistaxis
  - Extensive vascular supply to nose results in brisk epistaxis with trauma
- Change in appearance of the nose (displaced fracture)

Natural History

- Many nasal fractures remain untreated because of failure of diagnosis
- Untreated or poorly managed nasal fractures may result in residual cosmetic deformity and functional disability

Treatment

- Ice packs and elevation for initial treatment
- Non-displaced fractures do not require treatment
- Reduction and fixation indicated in any patient with cosmetic deformity or functional compromise
- Reduction may be closed or open
- Best time for reduction is first 3 hours after injury
  - Otherwise wait 7 to 10 days for edema to resolve

Prognosis

- Good with timely diagnosis and optimal treatment

Selected References

1. Rhea JT et al: The Face. Radiology of Skeletal Trauma. Ed by Rogers LF. Churchill Livingstone, Philadelphia 3rd ed. Vol 1:313-75, 2002
2. Rohrich RJ et al: Nasal fracture management: Minimizing secondary nasal deformities. Plast Reconstr Surg 106:266-73, 2000
3. Rhea JT et al: Helical CT and three-dimensional CT of facial and orbital injury. Radiol Clin North Am 37:489-513, 1999

Zygomatic Complex Fracture

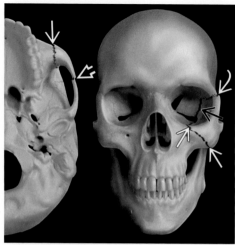

Zygoma complex fracture drawing. (Curved arrow) indicates zygomatico-frontal fracture. (Black arrow) indicates zygomatico-sphenoid fracture. (White arrows) indicate zygomatico-maxillary fractures. (Open arrow) indicates zygomatico-temporal fracture.

Key Facts
- Synonym(s): ZMC-fracture, zygoma fracture, tripod fracture, trimalar fracture, cheekbone fracture
- Definition: Fracture-dislocation of the zygoma bone
- Classic imaging appearance
  - Zygoma disarticulated from adjacent bones
- Other key facts
  - Second most commonly fractured facial bone
  - Usually caused by a blow to the side of the face
  - Pain, visual changes, cosmetic defects, difficulty opening mouth
  - CT is preferred imaging technique
  - Treatment with open reduction and fixation

Imaging Findings
General Features
- Best imaging clue: Zygoma disarticulated from adjacent bones
- Anatomy Findings
  - Anterior projection of zygoma forms the cheekbone or malar eminence
  - Zygoma articulates with four bones
    - Medially by the maxillary bone
    - Superiorly by the frontal bone
    - Posteriorly by greater wing of sphenoid bone
    - Laterally from the zygomatic process of the temporal bone
- Other generic features
  - Displaced fractures involve
    - Inferior orbital rim and orbital floor
    - Anterior and posterior-lateral walls of the maxillary sinus
    - Zygomaticofrontal suture
    - Zygomatic arch

Zygomatic Complex Fracture

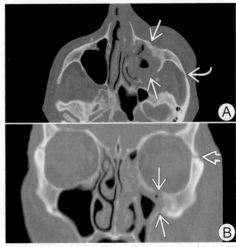

Zygoma complex fracture. (A) Axial CT scan shows zygomatico-maxillary fractures (arrows) involving anterior and posterior walls of maxillary sinuses. Curved arrow indicated zygomatico-temporal fracture. (B) Coronal CT shows zygomatico-maxillary fractures (arrows) and zygomatico-frontal fracture (open arrow).

Plain Film Facial Findings
- Opacification of ipsilateral maxillary sinus
- Ipsilateral orbital emphysema
- Zygoma disarticulated from maxillary, frontal, sphenoid and temporal bones
- Zygoma often displaced posterior and inferiorly

CT Findings
- Orbital floor fracture
- Inferior orbital rim fracture
- Fractures of anterior and posterior-lateral walls of maxillary sinus
- Fracture of zygomatic arch
- Disruption of zygomatico-frontal suture
- Disruption of zygomatico-sphenoid suture

Imaging Recommendations
- Plain film facial series
  - Composed of PA, lateral, base, Water's, Caldwell and Towne's views
- Non-contrast CT with 1.25 mm slices and routine coronal and sagittal reformations
  - Optimal imaging technique for suspected zygoma complex fracture

Differential Diagnosis
Soft Tissue Injury of Cheek
- Edema and hemorrhage but no fracture on plain films or CT
Orbital Blowout Fracture
- Similar orbital/ocular clinical findings and an orbital floor fracture
  - No orbital rim fracture
  - No other components of zygoma complex fracture

Zygomatic Complex Fracture

Pathology
Genera
- General Path Comments
  - Zygoma bone fractures and disrupts at articulations with maxillary, frontal, temporal and sphenoid bones
  - Many be associated with other facial fractures
  - 20% have an associated ocular injury
- Etiology-Pathogenesis
  - Mechanism usually a blow to the side of the face
  - Blow may result from a motor vehicle collision (80%), assault, fall, or sports-related injury
    - Moderate blows produces non-displaced or minimally displaced fractures
    - Severe blows produce displaced and comminuted fractures
- Epidemiology
  - Second most commonly fractured facial bone
  - Majority occur in men during their third decade

Classification
- No universally accepted classification system
- Fractures are classified on the basis of:
  - Degree of comminution; whether or not compound; site of the fractures; degree of displacement of fracture fragments; degree of rotation of fracture fragments

Clinical Issues
Presentation
- Pain, visual changes, cosmetic defects, difficulty opening mouth
  - Periorbital ecchymosis; subconjunctival hematoma; infraorbital nerve anesthesia; inferior orbital rim step-off on palpation; limitation of eye movements if inferior rectus muscle entrapped; flattening of the cheekbone; facial asymmetry; trismus; displaced fractures can limit movement of mandible

Treatment
- Non-displaced or minimally displaced fracture
  - Conservative management, antibiotics, no nose-blowing
- Displaced, comminuted, unstable or potentially unstable fracture
  - Open surgical reduction with rigid miniplate fixation & orbital floor repair
  - Surgery should be performed immediately or within 5 days
  - Closed reduction less commonly performed today

Prognosis
- Good prognosis with successful reduction and fixation
- Poorly reduced fractures may result in persistent diplopia, enophthalmos, exophthalmos, malunion, significant cosmetic deformity, persistent pain limitation of mandibular movements or a sensory or motor deficit

Selected References
1. Rhea JT et al:The Face. Radiology of Skeletal Trauma. Ed by Rogers LF. Churchill Livingstone, Philadelphia 3rd ed. Vol 1:315-75, 2002
2. Strong EB et al: Zygoma complex fracture. Facial plast surg 14:105-115, 1998
3. Covington DS et al: Changing patterns in the epidemiology and treatment of zygoma fractures: 10-year review. J Trauma 37:243-8, 1994

Zygomatic Arch Fracture

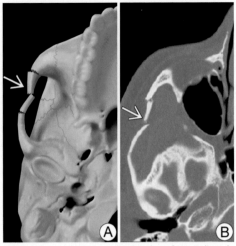

Zygomatic arch fracture. (A) Drawing showing three fracture lines (arrow) in the zygomatic arch with a V-shaped orientation of the medially displaced fracture fragments. (B) Axial CT scan showing three fracture lines (arrow) and a V-shaped orientation of the slightly depressed zygomatic arch fragments.

Key Facts
- Synonym: Zygomaticotemporal arch fracture
- Definition: Fracture of the zygomatic arch
- Classic imaging appearance
  - Three zygomatic arch fracture lines with fragments in a V-shaped configuration
- Other key facts
  - Represents 10-16% of zygoma fractures
  - Due to a blow to the side of the face by a small hard object
  - Patients present with regional pain, flattening of side of face and difficulty opening and closing mouth
  - Best shown on plain film base view, or axial CT
  - Treat with surgical restoration of the arch

Imaging Findings
Best Imaging Clue
- Fracture lines across the zygomatic arch
- Anatomy
  - Zygomatic arch is composed of the zygomatic process of the temporal bone and temporal process of the zygoma bone
  - The arch curves laterally over the temporalis muscle and coronoid process of the mandible
  - The arch also serves as the origin of the masseter muscle which attaches inferiorly to the lateral surface of the mandible
Plain Film Findings
- Base (submentovertical) view will best show zygomatic arch fractures
  - Base view may difficult to obtain in many trauma patients
- Arch fractures less well shown on Water's view
- See depression and/or displacement of arch fragments

Zygomatic Arch Fracture

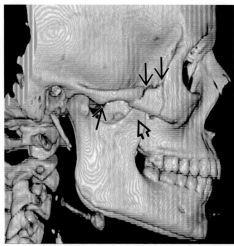

Zygomatic arch fracture. Right side view, 3D CT reformation of patient. Zygomatic arch fracture lines (arrows). Note relationship between coronoid process (open arrow) of mandible and overlying zygomatic arch. It is apparent why mandibular movements are impaired with zygomatic arch fractures.

CT Findings
- Zygomatic arch fractures best shown on axial slices
  - See three fractures of the zygomatic arch in a V-shaped configuration
- Fractures also well shown on 3D reformations

Imaging Recommendations
- Plain film facial series
  - Study base and Water's views for fractures of the zygomatic arch
- Facial CT is procedure of choice for zygoma fractures
  - 1.5 mm axial slices with coronal and sagittal reformations
  - Review axial slices for fracture lines in arch
  - Perform 3D reformations for positive cases to show displaced fractures
  - Review soft tissue windows for associated soft tissue injuries

Differential Diagnosis

Zygoma Complex Fracture
- CT shows additional fractures of the zygoma bone at the zygomatico-maxillary suture, zygomatico-frontal suture and zygomatico-sphenoid suture

Mandible Condyle or Mandible Ramus Fracture
- Patient will also have pain in region of temporomandibular joint and zygomatic arch as well as have difficulty opening and closing mouth
- Plain films or CT will shown mandible fracture rather than zygomatic arch fracture

Pathology

General
- General Path Comments
  - Based on force of blow, injuries range from mild bowing

Zygomatic Arch Fracture

- o When comminuted, usually three arch fractures with medial displacement of fracture fragments
- Etiology-Pathogenesis
  - o Usually the result of a direct blow to the side of the face by a small hard object
  - o Often resulting from an assault
- Epidemiology
  - o Most common isolated fracture of the zygoma
  - o Represents 10-16% of zygoma fractures
  - o More common in males

Clinical Issues
Presentation
- Regional pain over zygomatic arch
- Edema and hemorrhage over zygomatic arch
- Flattening of ipsilateral side of face
- Limited mandibular movements due to direct mechanical impingement of coronoid process of mandible against the displaced zygomatic arch
- Palpation of zygomatic arch step defects or contour abnormalities

Treatment
- Reconstruction of zygomatic arch with surgical reduction and fixation
- Various surgical approaches are directed at elevating fragments and restoring integrity of the arch

Prognosis
- Good prognosis with timely diagnosis and successful surgical repair
- Complications of surgery including bleeding and infection
- Unsatisfactory reduction can result in cosmetic and functional deficits
- A depressed arch can interfere with anterior and posterior excursions of the mandible

Selected References
1. Rhea JT et al: The face. Radiology of Skeletal Trauma. Ed by Rogers LF. Churchill Livingstone, Philadelphia 3rd ed, vol 1: 315-75, 2002
2. Covington DS et al: Changing patterns in the epidemiology and treatment of zygoma fractures: 10-year review. J Trauma 37:243-8, 1994
3. Zingg M et al: Classification and treatment of zygomatic fractures: 1,025 cases. J Oral Maxillofac Surg 50:778-790, 1992

Naso-Orbito-Ethmoid Fracture

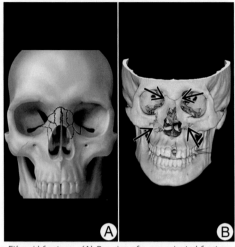

Naso-Orbito-Ethmoid fracture. (A) Drawing of a comminuted fracture of the naso-orbito-ethmoidal complex. (B) 3D CT reformation a naso-orbito-ethmoid fracture. Note the posterior displacement of the naso-orbito-ethmoid complex (arrows) and involvement of the medial orbits. Patient also lost an incisor tooth.

Key Facts
- Synonym(s): NOE fracture, naso-ethmoid fracture, naso-orbito-ethmoidal fracture
- Definition: Fracture of the naso-orbito-ethmoid (NOE) complex
- Classic imaging appearance
  - Comminuted and posteriorly displaced fractures of the NOE complex
- Other key facts
  - Challenging facial injury due to complexity of anatomical and functional components
    - Medial canthus tendon disruption
    - Nasolacrimal system injury
    - Intraorbital injuries
  - CT is imaging procedure of choice; plain films underestimates injury
  - Treatment usually requires open reduction and fixation

Imaging Findings
General Features
- Best imaging clue
  - Comminuted fractures of the nasal bones, frontal processes of maxillae, anterior-medial walls of maxillary sinuses and medial walls of the orbits
  - Fracture fragments displaced posteriorly into the ethmoid sinuses and orbits
- Anatomy
  - NOE complex represents the confluence of facial bones that separates the nasal, orbital and cranial cavities
  - Nasal, frontal, maxillary, ethmoid, lacrimal and sphenoid bones all contribute to the NOE complex

Naso-Orbito-Ethmoid Fracture

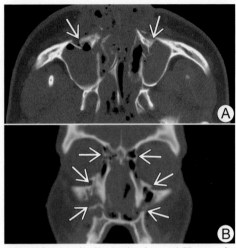

Naso-orbito-ethmoid fractures (A, B). Axial and coronal CT scans of patient in (A)
Axial scan shows fracturing of the anterior complex (frontal processes of maxillae)
(arrows) with posterior displacement of fragments. (B) Coronal scan shows fracturing
at the margins of the naso-orbito-ethmoid complex (arrows).

Plain Film Findings
- Plain film facial series of limited value in diagnosis
- Generally not able to characterize the NOE injury
- Show secondary findings of opacified maxillary and ethmoid sinuses

CT Findings
- Can show all components of, and correctly identify NOE fracture
- Clearly depicts position and orientation of fracture fragments
- Can show associated orbital soft tissue injuries
- Can show other associated facial fractures

Imaging Recommendations
- CT is procedure of choice; plain films underestimate this injury
- Non-contrast face CT scan with 1.5 mm slices from above frontal sinuses to below the mandible
- Routine coronal and sagittal reformations of the entire face

Differential Diagnosis

Nasal Fracture
- Fractures only of nasal bones, frontal processes of maxillae and anterior nasal spines of the maxilla
- The remainder of the NOE complex including the medial walls of the orbits remain intact

LeFort II Fracture
- Anterior components of LeFort II fracture similar to NOE
- In contrast, the LeFort II Fracture also extends posteriorly, fracturing the posterior-lateral walls of maxillary sinuses and the pterygoid plates

Naso-Orbito-Ethmoid Fracture

Pathology
Generale
- General Path Comments
  - Most NOE fractures comminuted with fragments posteriorly displaced
  - Medial canthal tendons are often disrupted resulting in traumatic telecanthus
  - Injuries to lacrimal apparatus may occur
- Etiology-Pathogenesis
  - A direct frontal force to the central midface
  - Motor vehicle accidents most common cause
  - Assaults second most common cause
- Epidemiology
  - Incidence in motor vehicle collisions is decreasing
    - May be related to increased use of air bags

Types
- Telescoped Type
  - The NOE complex is displaced posterior as a unit
- Comminuted Type
  - Extensive comminution with lateral spreading of fracture fragments

Clinical Issues
Presentation
- Obscuration of central facial bone architecture
- Soft tissue swelling, ecchymosis, hematoma
- Traumatic telecanthus
- Palpation may reveal mobile bony fragments, step-offs or crepitus

Natural History
- Untreated or poorly managed fractures will result in cosmetic deformity and functional disruption

Treatment
- Initial treatment includes patient stabilization and management of airway obstruction and excessive bleeding
- Definitive treatment with surgical reduction and fixation
  - Reduced openly by coronal scalp flap or directly though local incisions
  - Fixation with microplates
- When assocated with traumatic telecanthus, medial canthal tendons need to be reattached to prevent cosmetic deformity

Prognosis
- Prognosis good with timely CT diagnosis and optimal surgical reduction and fixation
- Prognosis affected by extent of fracture comminution, extent of fracture displacement, functional disruption and presence of related injuries

Selected References
1. Rhea JT et al: The Face. Radiology of Skeletal Trauma. Ed by Rogers LF. Churchill Livingston, Philadelphia, 3rd ed. Vol 1:315-75, 2002
2. Rhea JT et al: Helical CT and three-dimensional CT of facial and orbital injury. Radiol Clin North Am 37:489-513, 1999
3. Heine RD et al: Naso-orbital-ethmoid injury: Report of a review of the literature. Oral Surg Oral Med Pathol 69:542-9, 1990

Maxillary Sagittal Fracture

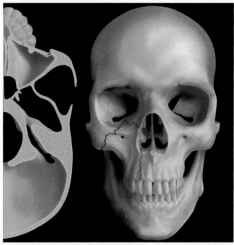

Maxillary sagittal fracture drawing. Fracture of anterior wall of right maxillary sinus with extension into orbital rim and floor due to a blow to the right midface.

Key Facts
- Synonym: Maxillary sinus fracture
- Definition: Fracture of one maxilla in the sagittal plane
- Classic imaging appearance
  - Fracture involves anterior-lateral wall of a maxillary sinus
  - May involve inferior orbital rim, orbital floor, frontal process of maxilla
- Other key facts
  - A type of isolated, unilateral maxillary fracture
    - Other isolated maxillary fractures include orbital rim fracture, orbital floor fracture and frontal process of maxilla fracture
  - Due to a direct blow to either right or left midface
  - Less common maxillary fracture than LeFort fractures
    - LeFort fractures represent bilateral maxillary fractures
  - Fracture may be linear, or may be comminuted and depressed

Imaging Findings
General Features
- Best imaging clues
  - Opacification of involved maxillary sinus
  - Anterior-lateral wall fracture of a maxillary sinus
- Anatomy
  - Paired maxillary sinuses prone to trauma because of they involve large areas of the face and have thin walls
  - Fracture of one maxillary sinus may be isolated or part of a more complex fracture
  - Anterior-lateral wall fracture is most common isolated maxillary fracture
Plain Film Facial Series
- Opacification of, or air-fluid level in involved maxillary sinus
- Orbital and subcutaneous emphysema
- Anterior-lateral wall fracture may be difficult to show on plain films

Maxillary Sagittal Fracture

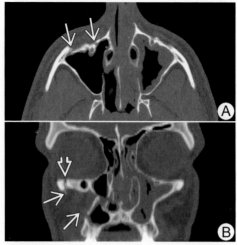

Maxillary sagittal fracture. (A) Axial CT scan shows a posteriorly depressed fracture (arrows) of the anterior wall of right maxillary sinus. (B) Coronal CT reformation shows medial displacement of the lateral wall (arrows) and extension of fracture into the inferior orbital rim (open arrow).

<u>CT Findings</u>
- CT excellent for showing fractures of the anterior-lateral wall of a maxillary sinus
- CT can differentiate between sinus opacification only and sinus opacification due maxillary sinus fracture
- CT will show all fracture lines, as well as the position and alignment of fracture fragments
- CT will show associated orbital emphysema, subcutaneous emphysema, and injury to orbital contents

<u>Imaging Recommendations</u>
- Plain film facial series for evaluation of this fracture is usually not adequate for diagnosis
  - Anterior-lateral wall fractures may show on Towne's or base views
- Perform non-contrast facial CT with 1.25mm slices and routine coronal and sagittal reformations

Differential Diagnosis
<u>LeFort Fractures</u>
- LeFort fractures represent bilateral maxillary fractures
  - Maxillary sagittal fracture is a unilateral maxillary fracture
- Differentiate with CT

Pathology
<u>General</u>
- General Path Comments
  - Fracture of anterior-lateral wall of a maxillary sinus which may extend into orbital rim and orbital floor

- May be associated with orbital emphysema, maxillary sinus hemorrhage and injury to orbital contents
- Etiology
  - Direct blow to the right or left midface with a small object
  - Site of blow usually directly overlying anterior wall of maxillary sinus
- Epidemiology
  - Maxillary fractures more common in 2nd to 3rd decade males
  - Maxillary blows less common than blows to the more prominent zygoma, nasal bones or mandible
  - Maxillary saggital fracture less common than LeFort fractures

Classification
- Maxillary fractures
  - Bilateral maxillary fractures
    - LeFort fractures
  - Unilateral maxillary fractures
    - Maxillary sagittal fracture
    - Orbital rim fracture
    - Orbital floor fracture
    - Frontal process of maxillary fracture

Clinical Issues

Presentation
- Plain, swelling, hemorrhage, epistaxis
- Crepitus due to subcutaneous emphysema
- Step-defect along inferior orbital rim with rim fracture
- Enophthalmus with displaced orbital floor fracture

Treatment
- Non-displaced fractures treated conservatively
- Displaced fractured may require surgical reduction and fixation

Prognosis
- Good prognosis with correct diagnosis and optimal treatment

Selected References
1. Rhea JT et al: The Face. Radiology of Skeletal Trauma. Ed by Rogers LF. Churchill Livingstone, Philadelphia, 2002
2. Muzaffar AR et al: Maxillary reconstruction: Functional and aesthetic considerations. Plast Reconstruc Surg. 104:2172-83, 1999
3. Werther JR: Fixation of sagittal fractures of the maxilla. Plast Reconstr Surg. 87(1):198-9, 1991.

LeFort I Fracture

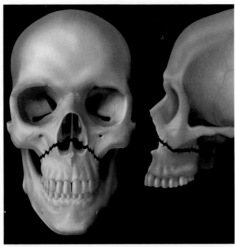

LeFort I fracture drawing. Note horizontal fracture line transversing lower maxillae, just above teeth roots. Fracture line extends posteriorly, and exits through pterygoid plates of sphenoid. Hard palate with maxillary teeth becomes freely moveable.

Key Facts
- Synonym: LeFort I maxillary fracture, LeFort I midface fracture
- Definition: Transmaxillary fracture
- Classic imaging appearance
  - Transverse (horizontal) fracture of the inferior maxillae, involving the anterior, lateral, medial and posterior walls of maxillary sinuses, the nasal septum and the pterygoid plates of the sphenoid
- Other key facts: Originally described by French physician Rene LeFort who identified lines of weakness in the face by traumatizing cadaver heads
  - LeFort fractures are among the most severe seen in the face and are associated with high energy trauma
  - LeFort I fracture represents a horizontal splitting of maxillae above hard palate
  - LeFort I fracture is most common LeFort fracture
  - Produces a floating & freely moveable hard palate

Imaging Findings
General Features
- Best imaging clue: Bilateral opacified maxillary sinuses, horizontal fracturing of lower maxillae above the hard palate
Plain Film Facial Series
- Will show opacification of both maxillary sinuses
- May show horizontal fracture across the maxillae
  - Water's and Caldwell views may show an interruption (fracture) of inferior aspects of both lateral walls of maxillary sinuses
  - Lateral view may show fractures of anterior and posterior walls of maxillary sinuses, with posterior extension of fracture through pterygoid plates

LeFort I Fracture

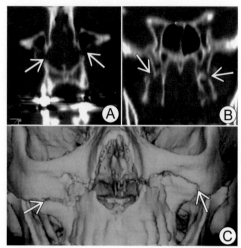

LeFort I fracture. (A) Anterior coronal CT reformation shows horizontal fx line (arrows) in lower maxillae above hard palate. (B) Posterior coronal reformation shows fracture line (arrows) extending through pterygoid plates. (C) 3D CT shows fracture line (arrows) with posterior displacement of hard palate fragment.

<u>CT Findings</u>
- Facial CT axial slices may only show a fracturing of inferior aspects of maxillary sinuses
- LeFort I fracture line best shown, and LeFort I fracture best confirmed on coronal and sagittal CT reformations
- CT may show bilateral maxillary sinus opacification or air-fluid levels

<u>Imaging Recommendations</u>
- Plain films may only show marked facial swelling with maxillary sinus opacification and may not adequately visualize the fracture
  - Water's Caldwell, Towne's, base and lateral views of the face
- CT is the ideal imaging modality for LeFort I fractures
  - Face CT with 1.25 mm axial slices
  - Routine coronal and sagittal reformations
  - 3D reformations if fracture fragments are displaced

Differential Diagnosis

<u>Maxillary Sagittal Fracture</u>
- This is a unilateral maxillary fracture

<u>LeFort II Fracture</u>
- Like a LeFort I fracture, the LeFort II fracture also involves the anterior-lateral walls of the maxillary sinuses but the LeFort II extends vertically to involve the inferior rims, floors and medial walls of the orbits and disrupts the naso-frontal sutures

Pathology

<u>General</u>
- General Path Comments

LeFort I Fracture

- o All LeFort fracture involve midface and produce freely floating segments of midface
- o All Le Fort fractures extend from front of face to back, involving pterygoid plates of sphenoid
- Etiology
  - o LeFort fractures usually result from high energy blunt trauma
    - Typical mechanisms include motor vehicle collisions, altercations, falls and sport-related injuries
  - o LeFort I fractures result from a direct horizontal blow to lower face
    - In a motor vehicle collision may caused by the steering wheel striking the face just under the patient's nose
    - Causes a shearing off of the hard palate and alveolar process
- Epidemiology
  - o LeFort fractures accounts for 6-25% of facial fractures
  - o More common in males in the 2nd and 3rd decade
  - o LeFort I is the most common LeFort fracture

Staging or Grading Criteria
- LeFort Fractures Classified as
  - o LeFort I
    - Transmaxillary fracture, produces a floating hard palate, transverse fracture across the maxilla just above the maxillary tooth apices, and posteriorly through the pterygoid plates
  - o LeFort II
    - Subzygomatic or pyramidal fracture
    - Produces a floating maxilla (zygomas not included)
  - o LeFort III
    - Craniofacial fracture, craniofacial separation; produces a floating face; complete midface separation of face from the skull including both zygomas
  - o Variants of this classification are frequently encountered

Clinical Issues
Presentation
- Severe midface soft tissue swelling and ecchymosis, epistaxis, upper airway obstruction
- On physical examination a freely floating and movable hard palate with maxillary teeth may be detected

Treatment & Prognosis
- Patients may require urgent intervention for airway management and bleeding
- LeFort fractures are associated with significant cosmetic and functional sequellae which require treatment with surgical reduction and fixation
- Repair of simple LeFort fractures typically results in restoration of facial contours and function
- LeFort I fractures generally have a favorable prognosis

Selected References
1. Rhea JT et al: The Face. Radiology of Skeletal Trauma. Ed by Rogers LF. Churchill Livingstone, Philadelphia 3rd ed, vol 1, 315-75, 2002
2. Muzaffar AR et al: Maxillary reconstruction: Functional and aesthetic considerations. Plast Reconstruc Surg 104:2172-83, 1999
3. Rhea JT et al: Helical CT and three-dimensional CT of facial and orbital injury. Radiol Clin North Am 37:489-513, 1999

LeFort II Fracture

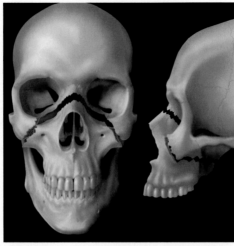

LeFort II fracture drawing. Note pyramid-shaped segment of moveable midface (maxillae, nasal bones). Fracture line extends down from naso-frontal sutures through medial walls, inferior rims and floors of orbits, through anterior walls of maxillary sinuses, under zygomas and out posteriorly through pterygoid plates.

Key Facts
- Synonym: LeFort II maxillary fracture, LeFort II midface fracture, pyramidal fracture
- Definition: Pyramid-shaped maxillary fracture, separating both maxillae & nasal bones as a unit from zygoma bones, medial walls of orbits and frontal bone
- Other key facts: Originally described by French physician Rene LeFort who identified lines of weakness in face by traumatizing cadaver heads
  - LeFort II fractures produces freely movable, pyramid-shaped segments of midface composed of maxillary teeth, hard palate & nose

Imaging Findings
General Features
- Best imaging clue: Bilateral opacified maxillary sinuses, fractures of anterior and posterior walls of maxillary sinuses, fractures of inferior orbital rims floors with fracture/disruption of naso-frontal sutures
Plain Film Facial Series
- Opacification of both maxillary sinuses and orbital emphysema
- May show pyramidal fracture line
  - Water's Caldwell views show fractures of lateral walls of maxillary sinuses with fractures of inferior orbital rims & floors
  - Lateral view may show disruption of naso-frontal sutures, fractures of anterior & posterior walls of maxillary sinuses, & fractures of pterygoid plates
CT Findings
- CT axial slices of face show characteristic fractures of anterior & posterior walls of maxillary sinuses with extension into pterygoid plates

LeFort II Fracture

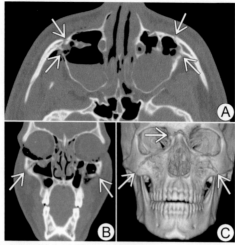

LeFort II fracture. (A) Axial CT shows bilateral fractures (arrows) of anterior and posterior walls of maxillary sinuses. (B) Coronal CT shows bilateral fractures (arrows) of anterior walls of maxillary sinuses extending up through orbital rims. (C) 3D CT shows LeFort II fracture line (arrows) margining midface segment.

- Coronal CT reformations show fractures of inferior rims and floors of orbits, as well as fractures of lateral walls of maxillary sinuses
- Bilateral maxillary sinus opacification or sinus air-fluid levels
- Orbital emphysema and subcutaneous emphysema

Imaging Recommendations
- Plain films may show marked facial swelling with maxillary sinus opacification and orbital emphysema, but may not adequately visualize extent of fracture
- CT is ideal imaging modality for LeFort II fractures
  - Face CT with 1.25 mm axial slices; routine coronal and sagittal reformations; 3D reformations if fracture fragments are displaced

Differential Diagnosis

Maxillary Sagittal Fracture
- This is a unilateral maxillary fracture
- LeFort II fractures are bilateral maxillary fractures

LeFort I Fracture
- Like a LeFort II fracture, the LeFort I fracture also involves anterior-lateral walls of maxillary sinuses
- However, LeFort II fracture extends vertically to involve inferior rims, floors and medial walls of the orbits and naso-frontal sutures

LeFort III Fracture
- Unlike LeFort II fracture, the LeFort III fracture is associated with bilateral zygomatic breaks separating the zygomatico-frontal sutures and disrupting the zygomatico-temporal arches

Naso-Orbito-Ethmoid Fracture
- Like NOE fracture the LeFort II fracture also involves anterior walls of maxillary sinuses, inferior rims of orbits and naso-ethmoid complex
- LeFort II fracture also extends posteriorly to back of face with fracture lines extending through pterygoid plates

LeFort II Fracture

Pathology
General
- General Path Comments: As defined by LeFort, LeFort fracture lines represent lines of weakness in face
  - All LeFort fracture involve midface & produce freely floating segments of midface
  - All LeFort fractures extend from front of face to the back, involving pterygoid plates of sphenoid
- Etiology: LeFort fractures usually result from high energy blunt trauma
  - Typical mechanisms include motor vehicle collisions, altercations, falls and sport-related injuries
  - LeFort II fractures result from a direct blow to lower or mid maxilla
- Epidemiology: LeFort fractures accounts for 6-25% of facial fractures
  - More common in males in 2nd and 3rd decade
  - LeFort fractures may occur in combination with other LeFort fractures or other facial fractures
    - Combined LeFort I and LeFort II fractures
    - Combined LeFort II and LeFort III Fractures
    - Combined LeFort II with a unilateral zygoma complex fracture

Staging or Grading Criteria
- LeFort Fractures Classified as
  - LeFort I: Transmaxillary fracture, produces a floating hard palate
  - LeFort II: Subzygomatic or pyramidal fracture
    - Produces a floating maxilla (zygomas not included)
  - LeFort III: Craniofacial fracture, craniofacial separation
    - Produces a floating face

Clinical Issues
Presentation
- Severe midface soft tissue swelling and ecchymosis, epistaxis, upper airway obstruction
- Peri-orbital swelling is seen with LeFort II fractures which involve
- Posterior protrusion of midface LeFort II segment give face a flattened appearance
- On physical examination a freely floating and movable midface segment including maxillary teeth, hard palate and nose

Treatment & Prognosis
- Patients may require urgent intervention for airway management & bleeding
- LeFort II fractures are associated with significant cosmetic and functional sequelae which require treatment with surgical reduction and fixation
- Repairs of simple LeFort fractures typically result in restoration of facial contour and function
- Repairs of complex LeFort II fractures may leave patients with residual cosmetic or functional deficits

Selected References
1. Rhea JT et al: The Face. Radiology of Skeletal Trauma. Ed by Rogers LF. Churchill Livingstone, Philadelphia 3rd ed. Vol 1:315-75, 2002
2. Muzaffar AR et al: Maxillary reconstruction: Functional and aesthetic considerations. Plast Reconstruc Surg 104:2172-83, 1999
3. Rhea JT et al: Helical CT and three-dimensional CT of facial and orbital injury. Radiol Clin North Am 37:489-513, 1999

LeFort III Fracture

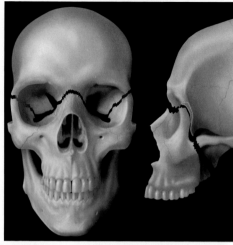

LeFort III Fracture Drawing. Facial bones are completely separated from the brain case or calvaria along LeFort III fracture line. The zygoma bones are separated from the frontal, sphenoid and temporal bones. The nasal bones, frontal processes of maxillae and medial orbital walls are separated from the frontal bone.

Key Facts
- Synonyms: LeFort III maxillary fracture, craniofacial disjunction
- Definition: Fracture which completely separates the facial bones from the skull or brain case (calvaria)
  - Traumatic craniofacial disjunction
- Classic imaging appearance
  - Line of fracturing extends through interface between facial and calvarial bones
- Other key facts
  - Originally described by French physician Rene LeFort who identified lines of weakness in the face by traumatizing cadaver heads
  - LeFort fractures are among the most severe seen in the face and are associated with high energy trauma
  - LeFort III is the most severe LeFort fracture
  - May be associated with a LeFort I, LeFort II or other facial fractures

Imaging Findings
General Features
- Best imaging clue: The facial bones, including the zygoma, maxillary, ethmoid, lacrimal and nasal bones are separated from the frontal, temporal and sphenoid bones
Plain Film Facial Series Findings
- Marked soft tissue facial swelling
- Water's and Caldwell views may show separation of zygomatico-frontal and naso-frontal sutures
- Lateral view may show separation of nasal bones and medial walls of the orbits from the frontal bone
CT Findings
- Axial and coronal CT shows separation of all facial bones from the

LeFort III Fracture

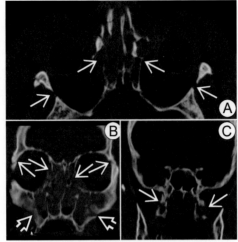

LeFort III fracture. (A) Axial CT shows line of craniofacial separation (arrows) Zygomas and nasal-ethmoid complex separated from sphenoid bone. (B, C) Coronal CT scans show LeFort III fracture line (arrows), extending posteriorly through pterygoid plates in C. Patient also has LeFort II Fracture (open arrows).

- o Zygomas separated from sphenoid at zygomatico-sphenoid sutures
- o Nasal bones and medial walls of the orbits separated from frontal bone at the naso-frontal sutures

Imaging Recommendations
- Plain films may underestimate extent of injury
  - o Facial swelling and hemorrhage obscure bony detail
  - o Difficult to obtain good quality plain films in patients with this injury
- CT will best show LeFort III fracture
  - o Non-contrast facial CT with 1.25 mm slices
  - o Obtain routine coronal and sagittal reformations
  - o Obtain 3D reformation for major displaced fracture fragments

Differential Diagnosis
LeFort II Fracture
- Both LeFort II and LeFort III fractures disrupt the naso-frontal sutures
- Unlike the LeFort III fracture, the LeFort II fracture extends inferiorly through inferior orbital rims, orbital floors and maxillary sinuses
- Unlike LeFort II fracture, the LeFort III fracture extends laterally through the zygomatico-frontal sutures separating the zygomas from the frontal and sphenoid bones

Pathology
General
- General Path Comments
  - o As defined by LeFort, LeFort fracture lines represent lines of weakness in the face
  - o All LeFort fracture involve the midface and produce freely floating segments of midface

LeFort III Fracture

- o All Le Fort fractures extend from the front of the face to the back, involving the pterygoid plates of sphenoid
- Etiology
  - o LeFort fractures usually result from high energy blunt trauma
    - Typical mechanisms include motor vehicle collisions, altercations, falls and sport-related injuries
- Epidemiology
  - o LeFort fractures accounts for 6-25% of facial fractures
  - o More common in males in the 2nd and 3rd decade
  - o LeFort fractures may occur in combination with other LeFort fractures or other facial fractures
    - Combined LeFort II and LeFort III Fractures
    - Combined LeFort III with a unilateral zygoma complex fracture

Classification
- LeFort I
  - o Transmaxillary fracture
  - o Produces a floating hard palate
- LeFort II
  - o Subzygomatic or pyramidal fracture
  - o Produces a floating maxilla (zygomas not included)
- LeFort III
  - o Craniofacial fracture, craniofacial separation
  - o Produces a floating face

Clinical Issues
Presentation
- Severe midface soft tissue swelling and ecchymosis
- Upper airway obstruction, epistaxis
- Epistaxis
- Flattening of the face due to posterior displacement of fragments
- Movement of the face relative to the skull
- CSF rhinorrhea
- Peri-orbital swelling with LeFort III fractures which involve the orbits
- Orbital involvement may result in enophthalmus, diplopia, extraocular muscle impairment, or ocular injury

Treatment
- Patients may require urgent intervention for airway management and bleeding
- LeFort III fractures are associated with significant cosmetic and functional sequellae which require treatment with surgical reduction and fixation

Prognosis
- Repairs of uncomplicated LeFort III fractures typically result in restoration of facial contour and function
- Repairs of complex LeFort III fractures with may leave patients with residual cosmetic or functional deficits

Selected References
1. Rhea JT et al: The Face. Radiology of Skeletal Trauma. Ed by Rogers LF. Churchill Livingstone, Philadelphia, 3rd edition, vol 1, pp 315-375, 2002
2. Muzaffar AR et al: Maxillary reconstruction: Functional and aesthetic considerations. Plast Reconstruc Surg 104:2172-83, 1999
3. Rhea JT et al: Helical CT and three-dimensional CT of facial and orbital injury. Radiol Clin North Am 37:489-513, 1999

Frontal Sinus Fracture

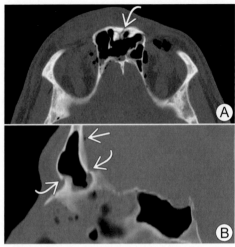

Frontal sinus fracture. (A) Axial CT through upper orbits shows fractures (curved arrow) of anterior wall of frontal sinuses. (B) Sagittal reformation shows fractures of the anterior and posterior walls (curved arrows). Straight arrow points to a tiny dot of pneumocephalus.

Key Facts
- Definition: Fracture of the frontal sinuses
- Classic imaging appearance
  - Fracture of anterior wall, posterior wall and/or floor of frontal sinuses with sinus opacification and/or air-fluid levels
- Other key facts
  - Among the least common facial fractures
  - Posterior wall fractures often associated with intracranial trauma

Imaging Findings
General Features
- Best imaging clue: Frontal sinus opacification and fractures
- Anatomy
  - Frontal sinuses are pyramid-shaped air spaces with an anterior wall, a posterior wall and a floor
    - Anterior walls are thickest
    - Posterior walls are thinner, separate frontal sinuses from brain
    - Floors are thinnest and separate frontal sinuses from orbits and ethmoid sinuses
    - The two frontal sinuses are separated by a midline septum

Plain Film Findings
- Sensitivity for diagnosing frontal fractures with plain films is low
- Plain films may show
  - Opacification of frontal sinuses
  - Air-fluid levels in frontal sinuses
  - Disruption of sinus walls
  - Intraorbital air with floor fractures
  - Pneumocephalus with posterior wall fractures

Frontal Sinus Fracture

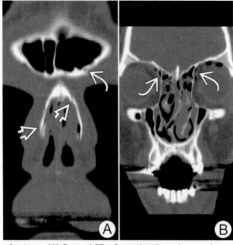

Frontal sinus fracture. (A) Coronal CT reformation through nose shows anterior wall left frontal sinus fracture (curved arrow) and nasal fractures (open arrows). (B) Coronal CT reformation through orbits shows fractures of base of frontal sinuses in superior-medial orbit (arrows). Note bilateral orbital emphysema.

CT Findings
- Highly accurate in diagnosing frontal sinus fractures
- Can identify extent of involvement of anterior wall, posterior wall and sinus floor fractures
- CT demonstration of fracture through base of sinus or extending into anterior ethmoid complex is suggestive of nasofrontal duct injury

Imaging Recommendations
- Plain films series with Water's, Caldwell, Towne's base and lateral views
- Non-contrast face CT scan with 1.25 mm slices
  - Review bone and soft tissue windows
  - Routine sagittal and coronal reformations

Differential Diagnosis
Other Facial Fractures
- Differentiate with facial CT

Pathology
General
- General Path Comments
  - Anterior wall fractures may be non-depressed, linear or depressed
  - Posterior wall fractures rarely isolated and may vertical or horizontal
    - Posterior wall fractures may be associated with intracranial injury
    - May be associated with dural tears and CSF leak
  - Fracture of the floor may result from an orbital blow-out or blow-in mechanism
- Etiology
  - Frontal sinus fractures may result from low-velocity, high velocity,

- With high velocity or penetrating trauma usually both anterior and posterior walls are fractured
  - Usually caused by blunt trauma during a vehicle collision
    - Forehead strikes automobile windshield
    - Motorcycle or bicycle accident in which rider is thrown over handlebars striking forehead on pavement
- Epidemiology
  - Less common facial fracture
  - Accounts for 5-12% of all facial fractures

Classification
- Anterior wall fracture
  - Simple linear, simple depressed, compound linear, compound linear depressed, compound comminuted
- Posterior wall fracture
  - With or without anterior wall fracture may be simple linear, compound linear, compound and/or comminuted depressed
- Sinus floor fracture
  - May be associated with any of the above fractures or with a naso-orbito-ethmoid fracture

Clinical Issues
Presentation
- Laceration or gross depression overlying the frontal sinuses
- More than 50% will have associated orbital trauma
- High incidence of coma or unsciousness
- High incidence of other fractures of the face or skull

Natural History
- Depressed fractures of the anterior wall can result in cosmetic deformity
- Fractures of posterior wall can result in CSF leak and meningitis
- Long-term complications of a frontal sinus fracture include formation of a frontal sinus mucocele which may
  - Create pressure necrosis of the frontal bone
  - Present later with a brain abscess, subdural abscess or "Pott's puffy tumor" (frontal bone osteomyelitis)

Treatment
- Goals of treatment are cessation of CSF leak, prevention of posttraumatic infection and restoration of facial contours
- All patients initially given prophylactic antibiotics
- Non-displaced fractures may not require intervention if they do not involve the naso-lacrimal duct
- Displaced fractures generally require exploration and reduction

Prognosis
- Good prognosis with early diagnosis and optimal
- Poorly managed fractures may lead to osteomyelitis, CSF leak, mucopyocele, meningitis, brain abscess or cavernous sinus thrombosis

Selected References
1. Rhea JT et al: The Face. In: Radiology of Skeletal Trauma. Ed by Rogers LF. Churchill Livingstone, Philadelphia, 3rd edition, vol 1 pp 315-375, 2002
2. Gerbino G et al: Analysis of 158 frontal sinus fractures: Current surgical management and complications. J Craniomaxillofac Surg 28:133-39, 2000
3. Rhea JT et al: Helical CT and three-dimensional CT of facial and orbital injury. Radiol Clin North Am 37:489-513, 1999

Mandible Fracture

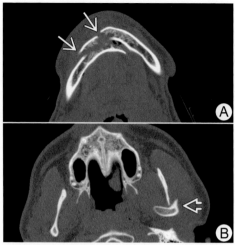

Mandible fracture. (A) Axial CT scan through symphysis shows fractures (arrows) of the right mandibular body. (B) Slightly higher axial CT through mandibular rami shows a fracture (open arrow) of the left mandibular condyle.

Key Facts
- Synonym(s): Jaw fracture
- Definition: Fracture of the bony mandible
- Classic imaging appearance
  o Fracture lines through mandible on plain films or CT
- Other key facts
  o One of the most common facial fractures
  o Usually caused by vehicular collisions and assaults
  o Multiple mandible fractures may occur
  o May be associated with other facial fractures

Imaging Findings
General Features
- Best imaging clue
  o Mandible fracture lines on plain film or CT
- Anatomy
  o Fractures classified by anatomic location within the mandible

Plain Film Mandible Series
- PA, lateral, Towne's and bilateral oblique plain films
- Will show nearly all mandibular fractures
- May be difficult to obtain in the multiple trauma patient

Panoramic Radiography Findings
- Gross screen for fractures
- Shows associated dental injuries
- Requires patient to be upright
  o Not possible for many trauma patients

CT Findings
- Non-contrast face CT will show all mandibular fractures as well as any associated facial fractures
- Will clearly display position and alignment of fracture fragments

Mandible Fracture

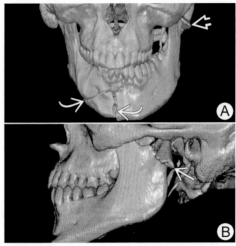

Mandible fracture. (A) Frontal view, 3D reformation, shows two fractures of the right mandible body (curved arrows); left condyle fracture fragment (open arrow). (B) Left side view, 3D reformation shows the subcondylar fracture (arrow) with subluxed condyle fragment.

- Will show associated soft tissue injuries
- Easy to perform in the multiple trauma patient
- Coronal and sagittal reformations should be routinely performed to visualize all fractures
- 3D reformations helpful for displaying displaced fracture fragments

Imaging Recommendations
- Screen with plain film mandible series or non-contrast CT
- CT should be performed if the plain films show a mandible fracture

Differential Diagnosis

Mandible Dislocation
- Mandible may be dislocated without fracture
- Patients present with an open mouth and severe mandible pain
- Patients unable to close the mouth
- Plain films and/or CT will show bilateral dislocation of the mandible condyles

General
- General Path Comments
  - Multiple mandible fractures may occur
    - Unilateral mandible fracture (70%)
    - Patients with 2 fractures (37%)
    - Patients with 3 fractures (9%)
  - When multiple fracture occur they are usually located on contralateral sides of the mandible
    - Common fracture is a bilateral fracture involving the symphyseal region on one side and the ramus on the other
  - Flail mandible occurs when a symphysis fracture is associated with bilateral subcondylar, ramus or angle fractures

Mandible Fracture

- The structural integrity of the mandible is lost and the tongue may fall back obstructing the airway
- Etiology
  - Vehicular collisions (43%); assaults (34%); falls (7%), work-related (7%); sports-related (4%)
- Epidemiology
  - Incidence by location
    - Body (29%); condyle (26%); angle (25%); symphysis (17%); ramus (4%); coronoid process (1%)

Staging or Grading Criteria
- Classification by anatomic region
  - Symphysis, parasympheseal, body, angle, ramus, condylar process, coronoid process, alveolar process
- Classification by fracture type
  - Simple or closed; compound or open; comminuted; greenstick; pathologic; multiple; impacted; atrophic

Pathology
- None relevant to this case

Clinical Issues
Presentation
- Patient may display facial lacerations, swelling and hematoma
  - Laceration under chin common with mandible fracture
- Mandible pain, areas of paresthesia or anesthesia
- Malocclusion of the teeth
- Deviation of mandible on opening mouth
- Abnormal mobility of portions of the mandible
- Step deformity on physical exam
- Intraoral or gingival tears

Treatment
- Closed reduction with arch bars, wires, loops
- Surgical open reduction

Prognosis
- Good with correct diagnosis and optimal treatment
- Complications may occur
  - Delayed union or nonunion
  - Infection
  - Malunion with improper alignment of healed bony segments
  - Ankylosis with intracapsular condyle fractures
  - Nerve injury
    - Inferior alveolar nerve and its branches are most commonly involved, resulting in numbness in the lower chin

Selected References
1. Rhea JT et al: The Face. Radiology of Skeletal Trauma. Ed by Rogers LF. Churchill Livingstone, Philadelphia, 3rd edition, vol 1 315-375, 2002
2. Ellis E III et al: Ten years of mandibular fractures: An analysis of 2137 injuries. J Oral Surg Oral Med Oral Pathol 59:120-9, 1985
3. Dolan KD et al: The radiology of facial fractures. Radiographics. 4:575-663, 1984

PocketRadiologist®

ER-Trauma

Top 100 Diagnoses

CERVICAL SPINE/NECK INJURY

Occipital Condyle Fracture

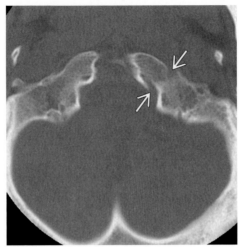

Axial CT scan shows a fracture of the left occipital condyle (arrows).

Key Facts
- Fracture easily overlooked or not visible on over 90% of plain films
- Plain radiographs will overlook about half of patients with acute craniocervical instability
- Associated cervical spine injury seen in about 32% of patients with occipital condyle fractures, especially C1 and C2 fractures
- Occur in about 4% of patients with significant head trauma
  - This fracture is indicator of high-energy trauma
- May be unilateral (77%) or bilateral
- Many occur in conjunction with subluxation of ipsilateral or contralateral condyle from the C1 lateral mass
- This injury is rare in children

Imaging Findings
General Features
- Other generic features: Mechanisms vary and include axial loading, rotational stress, and direct blows to the skull with extension of a fracture into the condyle usually from the occiput
- Anatomy: The alar ligaments run from the superolateral margin of the dens and attach to the occipital condyles; rotation puts the alar ligaments under stress and may result in an avulsion fracture
CT Findings
- Inferomedial avulsions are most frequent, accounting for 3/4 of occipital condyle fractures
- Compression fractures of the condyle may occur
- Associated subluxation of condyle from lateral mass of C1 frequent
Plain Film Findings
- Occipital condyles are very difficult to see on plain films
- Open mouth odontoid view provides best opportunity to see a condyle fracture
- Retropharyngeal soft tissue swelling

Occipital Condyle Fracture

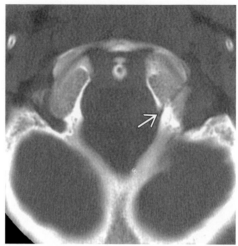

Same patient as previous page. The fracture is seen to extend obliquely through the condyle (arrow).

- Plain films are not sensitive to this injury (over 90% show nothing abnormal when condyle fracture is present)

Imaging Recommendations
- MR is best for assessment of ligaments
- Cervical spine CT is best to assess for fractures and should always include the occipitocervical junction

Differential Diagnosis
- None relevant to this case

Pathology
General
- Epidemiology
  ○ Occipital condyle fracture indicative of high-energy trauma

Staging or Grading Criteria
- Type 1: Stable, undisplaced fracture due to axial loading
- Type 2a: Stable, displaced fracture but ligaments intact
- Type 2b: Unstable, displaced fracture with ligamentous instability
- Type 3: Possibly unstable, avulsion fracture by the alar ligament from inferior medial aspect of condyle due to excessive rotation

Clinical Issues
Presentation
- Neck or occipital tenderness or pain, reduced head mobility, torticollis
- Depressed consciousness
- Injury to cranial nerves (i.e., hypoglossal nerve) occur in about 30% of patients with occipital condyle fracture
- Injury to brain stem or high cord
- Other craniocervical injury

Occipital Condyle Fracture

<u>Treatment</u>
- Need for surgical stabilization depends on stability of the injury
  - Unilateral fracture may be treated with halo fixation or Philadelphia collar
  - Bilateral joint injuries usually require surgery

Selected References
1. Momjian S et al: Occipital condyle fractures in children. Case report and review of the literature. Pediatr Neurosurg 38:265-70, 2003
2. Hanson JA et al: Radiologic and clinical spectrum of occipital ccondyle fractures: Retrospective review of 107 consecutive fractures in 95 patients. AJR Am J Roentgenol. 178:1261-8, 2002
3. Tuli S et al: Occipital condyle fracture. Neurosurgery. 41:368-76, 1997

Jefferson Fracture

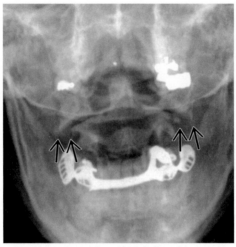

Open mouth odontoid view shows bilateral lateral offset of the articular masses of C1 relative to the articular masses of C2 (arrows). There is also a small fracture fragment from the left superior facet of the C2 vertebra.

Key Facts
- Synonym(s): Jefferson burst fracture
- Definition: Multiple fractures of the anterior and posterior C1 arch
- Classic imaging appearance: On plain film open mouth view there is bilateral lateral offset of the articular pillars of C1 relative to C2
  - In one series, the mean offset on each side was between 1 and 2 mm
- Other key facts
  - Mechanism of injury is axial loading
  - There must be fractures of both the anterior and posterior portions of the C1 ring
    - There may be one fracture anteriorly and two posteriorly
    - There may be two fractures anteriorly and two posteriorly
    - There may be unilateral anterior and posterior fractures
  - The transverse atlantal ligament may be torn leading to instability
    - If the sum of the offsets bilaterally is 7 mm or greater, the transverse ligament is assumed to be torn and the injury unstable
    - Measuring the offset may be done on the open mouth plain film on each side from the inferior lateral margin of the C1 pillar to the superior lateral margin of the C2 pillar
    - Measuring the offset may also be done from the coronal reformation
  - There is an association of C2 fractures with the Jefferson fracture
  - Other fractures of C1 include
    - Isolated posterior arch fracture due to hyperextension
    - Isolated articular mass fracture

Imaging Findings
<u>General Features</u>
- Best imaging clue: Bilateral lateral offset of the C1 articular masses relative to C2

Jefferson Fracture

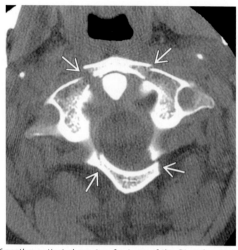

CT scan of another patient shows two fractures of the C1 arch anteriorly and two fractures posteriorly (arrows). The ADI appears to be normal, an unreliable finding in a supine scan.

- Anatomy: The transverse atlantal ligament attaches to the anterior portion of the C1 arch bilaterally and wraps posterior to the odontoid thus maintaining approximation of the odontoid to the anterior arch of C1

CT Findings
- Fractures in anterior and posterior portions of the C1 ring
- Coronal reformatted images show the lateral displacement of the C1 articular pillars
- The atlanto-dens interval (ADI) may be abnormal due to tear of the transverse atlantal ligament
  - ADI is the distance between the posterior margin of the anterior arch of C1 and the dens
  - Top normal ADI in adults is 3 mm and in pediatric patients is 5 mm
  - A normal ADI in an in-collar supine CT does not mean the transverse ligament is intact

MR Findings
- Ligamentous damage may be shown

Plain Film Findings
- Bilateral lateral offset of the lateral masses of C1 relative to the articular masses of C2 on the open mouth view
- Fractures of the C1 ring may be seen on the lateral or oblique views

Imaging Recommendations
- CT is the modality of choice to assess cervical spine fractures.
- CT parameters include 2.5 mm image thickness and spacing and a detector configuration which would allow reformations to 1.25 mm
- Sagittal and coronal reformations should always be obtained

Differential Diagnosis
- Bilateral fractures of the posterior arch of C1
  - This injury is due to hyperextension
  - There are associated type 2 dens fractures

Jefferson Fracture

- o There is no characteristic lateral displacement of the articular masses of C1 with only posterior arch fractures
- Normal variation
  - o If there are congenital areas of failure of ossification of the midline anterior and posterior arch of C1, there may be minimal (< 1 mm) bilateral lateral offset of the articular masses of C1
  - o On the lateral plain film, the equivalent of the spino-laminar line (anteriorly convex line of cortical bone at the junction of the spinous process and lamina) will be absent with a defect in the posterior arch of C1

Pathology
- None relevant to this case

Clinical Issues
Presentation
- Upper neck pain and tenderness
- Limited mobility of the head
- History of axial loading to the head

Treatment
- Surgical stabilization is necessary with unstable injury
- Stable injury may be treated with a halo or rigid collar for 10-12 weeks

Selected References
1. Prempe RC et al: Mid-line clefts of the atlas: A diagnostic dilemma. Spinal Cord. 40:92-3, 2002
2. Abuamara S et al: Posterior arch bifocal fracture of the atlas vertebra: A variant of Jefferson fracture. J Pediatr Orthop B. 10:201-4, 2001
3. Lee TT et al: Treatment of stable burst fracture of the atlas (Jefferson fracture) with rigid cervical collar. Spine. 23:1093-7, 1998

Atlanto-Occipital Subluxation

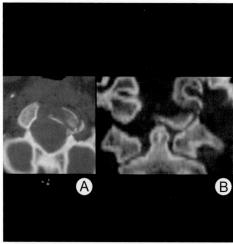

(A) Axial CT shows a fracture of the left occipital condyle. (B) Coronal CT reformation through the occipital – C1 articulation shows that this slightly comminuted fracture line on the left lies in the axial plane.

Key Facts
- Synonym(s)
  - Atlanto-occipital dislocation
  - Occipitovertebral dissociation
- Definition: Subluxation, dislocation or distraction of the occipital condyles from the superior articular surface of C1
- Classic imaging appearance: Alignment of the skull relative to the cervical spine is abnormal
- Other key facts
  - Dislocation my occur anteriorly or posteriorly and usually results in death due to damage to the brain stem (medulla)
  - Subluxation, partial "uncovering" of the joint surface, may be a survivable injury, but cord damage is frequent
  - Distraction is axial displacement of the head from the spine
  - Cranio-cervical ligamentous injury almost always leads to prevertebral hemorrhage
  - Children survive the injury more frequently than adults
  - Fracture of the occipital condyle occurs in over 15% of patients
  - Associated fracture of cervical vertebra may occur

Imaging Findings
General Features
- Best imaging clue: Abnormal alignment of occipital condyles relative to the superior articular facets of C1
- Anatomy
  - Ligaments
    - Inner layer: Paired alar, apical, cruciform and tectorial
    - Outer layer: Capsular, anterior and posterior atlanto-occipital, nuchal
  - Ligaments most important for maintaining stability: Tectorial and alar

Atlanto-Occipital Subluxation

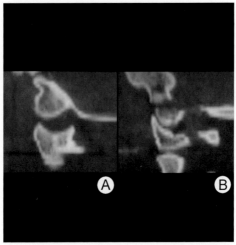

(A) Sagittal CT reformation through the right occipital condyle shows distraction and slight anterior subluxation. (B) Sagittal CT reformation through the left occipital condyle shows horizontal fracture with distraction through the site of fracture.

- o Ligaments allow flexion-extension and lateral bending but not rotation at the atlanto-occipital joints

CT Findings
- Abnormal alignment is best seen on sagittal and coronal reformations
  - o Joint widening and anterior or posterior displacement of the occipital condyles relative to C1 will be seen
  - o The basion-dens interval (BDI) and basion axial interval (BAI) will be abnormal
- Prevertebral soft tissues will usually demonstrate a taut anterior convexity

MR Findings
- Edema or disruption of ligamentous structures and brain stem injury may be seen

Plain Film Findings
- Measuring the BDI and BAI on the lateral view are useful since the mastoids may obscure the widened joint space or displacement at the condyle – C1 facet joint
  - o BDI is the shortest distance between the basion and dens
    - ▪ 12 mm is top normal
    - ▪ BDI is especially sensitive to distraction of occiput from C1
  - o BAI is the perpendicular distance between the basion and a line drawn through the posterior cortex of the body of C2 and extended upward
    - ▪ Normal range for the position of the basion relative to the line drawn is from 12 mm anterior to 4 mm posterior
    - ▪ BAI is especially sensitive to anterior or posterior displacement of the occiput relative to C1
- The joint space between the superior facet of C1 and the occipital condyle may appear widened on the lateral view if not obscured by the mastoid air cells

Atlanto-Occipital Subluxation

Imaging Recommendations
- MR best depicts ligamentous injury
- CT best depicts abnormalities of alignment and presence of fractures

Differential Diagnosis
Atlanto-Occipital Subluxation in Rheumatoid Arthritis
- Rare

Pathology
Staging or Grading Criteria
- Three forms of this injury are described based on the direction of displacement
  - o Anterior displacement of head relative to cervical spine
  - o Distraction of head relative to cervical spine
  - o Posterior displacement of head relative to cervical spine
    - More than half of these injuries are a combination of anterior displacement and distraction

Clinical Issues
Presentation
- Glasgow coma scale may be normal or abnormal
- Pain
- Limited motion of head
- Cranial nerve injury
- Vertebral artery injury due to stretching and thrombosis

Treatment
- Ligamentous instability would be an indication for surgical fusion

Prognosis
- Dislocations usually lead to instant death
- Survival, though with neurological impairment such as quadriplegia, is possible with mild distraction and subluxation

Selected References
1. Deliganis AV et al: Radiologic spectrum of craniocervical distraction injuries. Radiographics. 20:S237-50, 2000
2. Bloom AI et al: Fracture of the occipital condyles and associated craniocervical ligament injury: Incidence, CT imaging and implications. Clin Radiol. 52:198-202, 1997
3. Harris JH et al: Radiologic diagnosis of traumatic occipitovertebral dissociation: 2. Comparison of three methods of detecting occipitovertebral relationships on lateral radiographs of supine subjects. AJR Am J Roentgenol. 162:887-92, 1994

Atlanto-Axial Rotatory Fixation

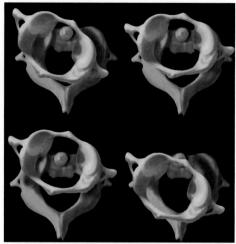

The position of C1 relative to C2 in the types of AARF is shown. Type 1 (A) appears rotated but is normal radiographically with symmetric anterior motion on one side and posterior motion on the other side. The other types demonstrate various abnormal positions of C1 relative to C2 as described below.

Key Facts
- Definition: Fixed rotation of C1 on C2 due to injury of the capsular ligaments or synovium at the facet joints of C1-2
  - The patient cannot voluntarily straighten out this rotation
- Classic imaging appearance: Two factors need to be assessed: Rotation of C1 on C2 and atlanto-dens interval (ADI)
  - Top normal rotation of C1 on C2 is 45 degrees as measured on the axial CT images
  - ADI may be measured on axial CT images or lateral reformation in the midline
    - Top normal ADI in adults is 3 mm; in children 5 mm
    - ADI may be "V shaped"; measure shortest distance
- Anatomy
  - Ligaments: Transverse atlantal, alar, accessory atlanto-axial, tectorial
  - Motion: About 45 degrees of rotation and 10 degrees of flexion/extension but no lateral bending
    - Flexion limited by tectorial ligaments
    - Extension and posterior translation limited by approximation of C1 arch against dens
    - Rotation limited by alar ligaments
    - Anterior translation limited by transverse atlantal ligaments

Imaging Findings
Plain Film Findings
- Best imaging clue: On an open mouth plain film view, there may appear to be overlap of the articular pillars of C1 and C2 on the same side, known as the "wink sign"
  - The contralateral side will appear to be of normal width
CT Findings
- Type 1 injury

Atlanto-Axial Rotatory Fixation

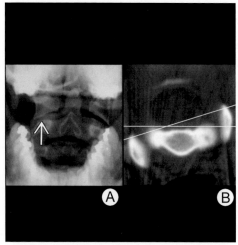

(A) On the open mouth view, there is overlap of the articular pillars of C1 and C2 on the right side. (B) Axial CT image shows about 30 degrees of rotation of C1 relative to C2. On other images the ADI was normal.

- o Normal amount of symmetric rotation of C1 on C2 with one side of C1 moving anteriorly and the other posteriorly
- o ADI is normal
- Type 2 injury
  - o Pivoting of the C1-2 articular pillars on one side and contralateral anterior subluxation of C1 relative to C2
  - o The ADI is abnormal
- Type 3 injury
  - o Bilateral asymmetric anterior subluxation of the pillars of C1 relative to C2
  - o The ADI is abnormal
- Type 4 injury
  - o Bilateral asymmetric posterior subluxation of the pillars of C1 relative to C2
  - o The dens may be absent or fractured
- Type 5 injury
  - o Unilateral dislocation and contralateral subluxation or bilateral dislocation of the facet joints
  - o The ADI is abnormal
  - o Bilateral dislocation requires about 65 degrees of rotation
  - o One side moves anteriorly and the other posteriorly

Imaging Recommendations
- This injury is best evaluated with CT

Differential Diagnosis
Torticollis
- Not synonymous with AARF
- Rotation of C1 on C2 due to muscle spasm
- No muscle spasm in AARF

Atlanto-Axial Rotatory Fixation

Pathology
- None relevant to this case

Clinical Issues
Presentation
- Neurological injury is rare, but may occur
- Vertebral artery injury may occur leading to brain damage

Selected References
1. Rhea JT: Rotational injuries of the cervical spine. Emergency Radiology 7:149-59, 2000
2. Wise JJ et al: Traumatic bilateral rotatory dislocation of the atlanto-axial joints: A case report and review of the literature. J Spinal Disord 10:451-3, 1997
3. Fielding JW et al: Atlanto-axial rotatory fixation: Fixed rotatory Subluxation of the atlanto-axial joint. J Bone Joint Surg Am 59:37-44, 1977

Odontoid Fracture

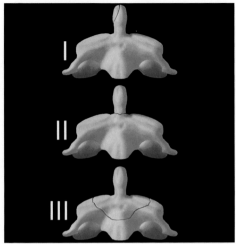

Type I is an avulsion from the superolateral aspect of the dens near the insertion of the alar ligaments. Type II is a transverse fracture through the base of the dens. Type III is a fracture that dips down into the body of C2 separating the dens and a fragment of the body from the remainder of the body.

Key Facts
- Synonym(s): Odontoid fracture and dens fracture are synonymous
- Definition: The odontoid of C2 is the axis about which C1 rotates
- Classic imaging appearance: Most frequent, over 60%, is the type II fracture; type I is rare
- Other key facts
  - Because the type II fracture is oriented in the axial plane, axial CT images or thick CT images may miss this fracture; thin images, coronal and sagittal reformations are needed
  - Mechanism can be flexion or extension leading to anterior or posterior displacement of the odontoid and possibly angulation through the site of fracture
  - Odontoid fractures are associated with C1 fractures
    - Jefferson fracture
    - Isolated anterior or posterior fractures of C1
    - Rare bilaterally posteriorly displaced atlanto-axial rotatory subluxation injury
  - Fracture may be comminuted with a vertical component through the odontoid

Imaging Findings
General Features
- Best imaging clue: Transverse lucency at base of odontoid on lateral view or sagittal or coronal reformations
- Anatomy
  - In children, a synchondrosis occurs between ossification centers of the dens and the body of C2; this rarely is injured and widened in trauma
  - The os terminale, a small separate ossification center, occurs at the tip of the dens in the midline

Odontoid Fracture

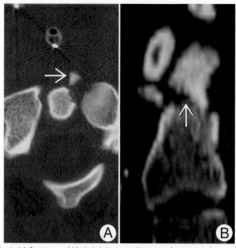

Type II odontoid fracture. (A) Axial image shows a fragment from the odontoid (arrow). (B) Sagittal image in the midline shows the transverse fracture at the base of the odontoid (arrow) typical of the type II fracture. The fracture fragment is seen anteriorly

CT Findings
- Type I fracture at supero-lateral aspect of the dens would be seen on axial or coronal images
- Type II fracture at base of dens may be very difficult to see on the axial images; is best seen on the sagittal reformation in the midline with multislice scanners
- Type III fracture is curvilinear convex caudad with the fracture entering the superior facets of C2 and dipping down into the C2 body

Other Modality Findings
- Plain film imaging may show the type III fracture entering the superior facets of C2 on the oblique views
- The lateral view best shows the type II fracture through the base of the odontoid

Imaging Recommendations
- CT rather than plain films should be used to evaluate patients with significant cervical spine trauma
- MRI may be done to better depict the status of the spinal cord and cervical nerve roots

Differential Diagnosis
Fractures of C2 Vertebral Body
- Coronally or sagittally oriented fractures located between odontoid and pars interarticularis

Pathology
- None relevant to this case

Odontoid Fracture

Clinical Issues
Presentation
- Patients may present only with pain
- Neurological findings are possible if the fracture is significantly displaced against the cord

Treatment
- Immobilization with halo fixation

Prognosis
- Outcome is very good if there is no initial neurological injury

Selected References
1. Castillo M et al: Vertical fractures of the dens. AJNR Am J Neuroradiol. 17:1627-30, 1996
2. Benzel EC et al: Fractures of the C2 vertebral body. J Neurosurg. 81:206-12, 1994
3. Anderson LD et al: Fractures of the odontoid process of the axis. J Bone Joint Surg. 56:1663, 1974

Hangman's Fracture

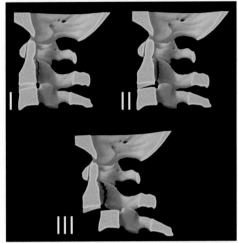

The severity of Hangman's fracture is variable. Type I: There are bilateral fractures involving pars interarticularis. Type II: There is also disruption of disc at C2-3. The body of C2 may angulate or may sublux. Type III: There is dislocation or disruption of articular facets of C2-3 in addition to the other findings.

Key Facts
- Synonym(s): Traumatic spondylolisthesis of the axis; fracture of the neural arch or ring of the axis
- Definition: Bilateral fracture of the pars interarticularis of C2
- Other key facts
  - One of the most common injuries of the cervical spine
  - Mechanism
    - Hyperextension, as in judicial hanging
    - Hyperflexion with axial loading
  - Frequency of types of Hangman's fracture: Type 1 > type 2 >type 3
    - Over half are type 1 fractures
  - Fracture line
    - May extend into the inferior or superior articular facet of C2
    - May extend into the posterior inferior aspect of the body of C2
  - Rarely the pars fracture may be unilateral
  - Associated C1 fractures are seen in about ¼ of patients with Hangman's fracture
  - May occur rarely in infants and children

Imaging Findings
General Features
- Anatomy
  - C2 does not have a pedicle
  - The anterior portion of the articular mass fuses with the body of C2; this region of fusion is analogous to the pedicle at other cervical levels
  - The articular mass at C2 is not quadrilateral in shape, as is true usually from C3 through C6; shape is more complex and elongated

Hangman's Fracture

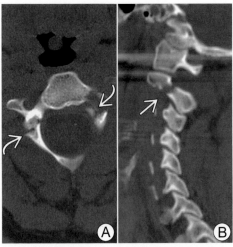

Hangman's fracture. (A) Axial CT image shows fractures just posterior to vertebral body in pars interarticularis (arrows). (B) Sagittal reformation through the articular facets shows the fracture on the left passing purely through the pars (arrow). The fracture through the right pars extended into the inferior articular facet.

- The superior facet of C2 is more horizontal than other cervical facets and lies in the same coronal plane as the odontoid
- The inferior facet of C2 is more posteriorly located adjacent to the superior facet of C3 and assumes the obliquity characteristic of other lower levels
  o The portion of bone between the superior facet and inferior facet of C2 is the pars interarticularis and is seen on a lateral view just posterior to the vertebral body

CT Findings
- The articular masses of C2 constitute the anterolateral portions of the neural arch on axial images
- Fractures will be seen involving this bone between the facets of C2
- Fractures may extend through the facet surfaces as they break the pars interarticularis
- The pars fractures are most easily appreciated on sagittal CT reformations

Plain Film Findings
- Nondisplaced pars fractures may be undetected on plain films
- Fracture of pars is seen on lateral view just posterior to the vertebral body
- The two pars may be exactly superimposed on lateral view
  o With patient tilt to one side, the superior cortex of the pars may be separated slightly in the vertical plane on lateral view, allowing detection of subtle fractures
- The oblique views best show the pars as the posterior superior margin of the C2-3 foramen
  o Fractures well seen on this view, including those that cross through the superior articular facet of C2

Hangman's Fracture

Imaging Recommendations
- CT is best at detecting fractures and alignment abnormalities
- Technique includes 2.5 mm image spacing and thickness with detector configuration on multislice set to allow 1.25 mm reformations
- MR is indicated with neurological signs and symptoms

Differential Diagnosis
- None relevant to this case

Pathology
Staging or Grading Criteria
- Type 1: Fractures of the pars interarticularis
- Type 2: Fracture of the pars plus disc injury at C2-3 allowing angulation of the body of C2 and dens or distraction with anterolisthesis of the body of C2
- Type 3: Fracture of the pars and disc injury plus disruption or dislocation of the C2-3 facet joints

Clinical Issues
Presentation
- Neck pain and tenderness
- Reduced head motion
- Possible cord damage

Treatment
- Traction needed prior to halo immobilization if there is significant (> = 12 degrees) angulation or distraction through the site of fracture in type 2
- More severe injuries may require surgical stabilization

Prognosis
- Extension of fracture into the transverse foramen may cause injury to the vertebral artery with thrombosis or rarely cerebellar embolization

Selected References
1. Vaccaro AR et al: Early halo immobilization of displaced traumatic spondylolisthesis of the axis. Spine. 27:2229-33, 2002
2. Parisi M et al: Hangman's fracture or primary spondylolysis: A patient and a brief review. Pediatr Radiol. 21:367-8 year
3. Mirvis SE et al: Hangman's fracture: Radiologic assessment in 27 cases. Radiology. 163:713-7, 1987

Unilateral Interfacetal Disloc.

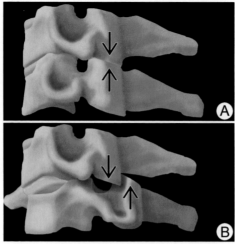

(A) The normal relationship involves apposition of the flat surfaces of the articular pillars. (B) In unilateral facet dislocation the articular pillar superior to the dislocated facet joint has moved anteriorly and dislocated in front of the articular pillar inferior to the facet joint. The convex surfaces of the articular pillars are apposed.

Key Facts

- Definition: Unilateral interfacetal dislocation (UID) consists of a unilateral malposition of the facet surfaces of a facet joint in which one articular pillar moves anteriorly and falls inferiorly relative to the pillar below, thus "locking" into this abnormal position
- Classic imaging appearance: Abnormal apposition of the articular pillars at any level with a rotational discrepancy of the spine above the level of UID relative to the spine below the level of UID is seen
- Other key facts
  - Fracture of the pillar that dislocated is a frequent occurrence
  - The contralateral side may sublux
  - Either ipsilateral fracture or contralateral subluxation can result in a lesser degree of rotational discrepancy than would be expected without these simultaneous abnormalities
  - UID is seen in about 10% of cervical spine fractures and dislocations
  - The most frequent level is at C5-6 and C6-7 although any level may be involved
  - C7-T1 may be the level of dislocation; thus it is imperative to always image down to T1 on a cervical spine examination
  - Simultaneous injury to the cervical spine above or below the level of the UID will occur in about 25% of patients

Imaging Findings

Plain Film Findings

- On the lateral view, the articular pillars are usually seen as quadrilateral shapes from C3 through C6; the dislocation of the facet surfaces will be apparent because the pillars do not stack on top of each other

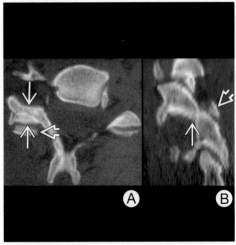

(A) On the axial image the flat surfaces of the pillars are separated (arrows) and the curved surfaces are apposed and overlap. There is also a fracture fragment (open arrow). (B) The sagittal reformation shows the dislocation (arrows) and a fracture fragment from the articular pillar (open arrow).

- There is anterolisthesis of the upper vertebral body on the lower, usually by less than half the width of the vertebral body
- All views show rotation of the spine above the level of injury relative to the spine below the level of injury
  - On lateral view the pillars may assume a "bowtie" appearance due to rotation above the level of injury
  - On oblique views the laminae are likened to "shingles on a roof" with the inferior margin of one being posterior to the superior margin of the lower lamina; in dislocation, there is interruption of this "shingles on a roof" appearance

CT Findings
- On axial images at the level of a facet joint, the pillars normally look like a hamburger bun with the flat surfaces apposed
  - In dislocation the curved surfaces of the pillars are apposed, and the flat surfaces are separated from each other
  - An axial image may show an "empty facet" which is an abnormal appearance and may be seen in either dislocation or subluxation of the joint
- Sagittal reformations through the articular pillars will show the dislocation and allow easy diagnosis of this entity

Imaging Recommendations
- CT rather than plain films should be used to evaluate patients with significant trauma
- UID is easily diagnosed at CT and associated fractures may not be visible on plain films
- MRI may be indicated to better depict the condition of the spinal cord and cervical nerve roots

Differential Diagnosis
• None relevant to this case

Pathology
• None relevant to this case

Clinical Issues
Presentation
• About 2/3 of patients with UID have radicular symptoms or neurological deficit

Selected References
1.   Rhea JT: Rotational injuries of the cervical spine. Emergency Radiology 7:149-59, 2000
2.   El-Khoury GY, et al: Imaging of acute injuries of the cervical spine: Value of radiography, CT, and MR imaging. AJR Am J Roentgenol 161:43-50, 1995
3.   Argenson C et al: Traumatic rotatory displacement of the lower cervical spine. Spine 13:767-73, 1988

Bilateral Interfacetal Disloc.

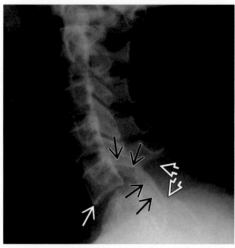

The lateral view shows widening of the interlaminar distance (open arrows) and anterolisthesis of the upper vertebra (white arrow). The facet surfaces are not apposed (black arrows) with the inferior facets of the upper vertebra located anterior and slightly inferior to the superior facets of the lower vertebra.

Key Facts
- Definition: Both articular pillars dislocate relative to their corresponding pillars at the level below
- Classic imaging appearance: Fanning posteriorly, anterolisthesis by ½ of more of the width of the vertebral body, and "locking" of the facets at the level of injury

Imaging Findings
Plain Film Findings
- Best imaging clue: Dislocation of the articular pillar facets seen on the lateral plain film
- Other generic features
  - The oblique plain films will show interruption of the "shingles on a roof" appearance of the laminae
  - No rotational discrepancy of the upper cervical spine on the lower is present
- Anatomy
  - Articular pillars are quadrilateral shaped structures from C3 to C6, which are held in place anteriorly by the pedicle and posteriorly by the lamina
  - The pillar of C2 is more complex in shape with wider separation of the superior and inferior facets (joint surfaces) in the horizontal plane
  - In cervical spine, only C2 has a pars interarticularis, the piece of bone between the articular facets
  - The C7 pillar usually is more complex in shape, extending further posterior than the other cervical pillars and having frequently an indentation along its superior surface
    - Indentation lines up with the posterior aspect of the articular pillars of the upper portion of the cervical spine

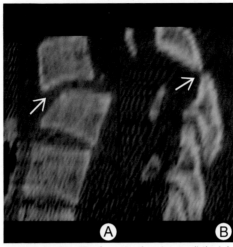

(A) In BID with sagittal midline CT reformation there is anterolisthesis by about 50% of the AP dimension of the vertebra (arrow). (B) Articular pillar dislocation in parasagittal CT reformation (arrow).

CT Findings
- Axial images
  - At the facet joint two pieces of bone normally should be seen
    - Anteriorly is the pillar from the vertebra below the joint
    - Posteriorly is the pillar from the vertebra above the joint
  - If three or more pieces of bone are seen, fracture dislocation should be suspected
  - Image through the facet joint should show the flat surfaces of the articular pillars apposed and the convex surfaces opposite each other, analogous to a hamburger bun
  - With dislocation, the convex surfaces are apposed and the flat surfaces are separated, analogous to a reversed hamburger bun
- Sagittal reformation
  - Through articular pillars shows anterior and inferior displacement of the pillar above relative to the pillar below
  - Through the midline shows anterolisthesis on the upper vertebra on the lower
- Fracture-dislocation may show less anterolisthesis than expected without fracture

Imaging Recommendations
- CT should be performed to assess bony fracture and subluxation or dislocation
- MRI may be performed to assess the spinal cord and ligaments

Differential Diagnosis
Subluxation of the Articular Pillars
- In subluxation there is partial "uncovering" of the apposing facet surfaces due to anterior motion on the upper articular pillar on the lower

- Perching of the articular pillars
  - When perched, the posterior inferior margin of the upper pillar impinges on the anterior superior margin of the lower pillar
    - Perched pillars may not reduce without traction

Pathology
- None relevant to this case

Clinical Issues
Presentation
- The degree of ligamentous injury to all three columns results in an unstable injury
- Quadriplegia is very frequent
- Presentation is variable with complete or incomplete spinal cord injury

Treatment
- Surgical decompression, reduction, and stabilization

Prognosis
- Partial recovery may be seen in some patients, although prognosis is poor with BID

Selected References
1.   Van Goethem JW et al: Cervical spine fractures and soft tissue injuries. JBR-BTR. 86:230-4, 2003
2.   Wang MY et al: Minimally invasive lateral mass screws in the treatment of cervical facet dislocations: technical note. Neurosurgery. 52:444-7; discussion 447-8, 2003
3.   Holmes JF et al: Variability in computed tomography and magnetic resonance imaging in patients with cervical spine injuries. J Trauma. 53:524-9, 2002

Teardrop Fractures

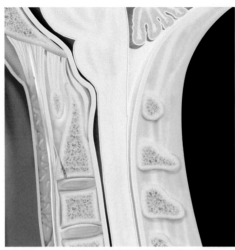

In a teardrop fracture, a small triangular fragment from the inferior anterior portion of the vertebral body is pulled off by the anterior longitudinal ligament or is avulsed by impaction on the vertebral body below the fracture.

Key Facts

- Definition: Triangular shaped fragment as seen on lateral view occurs at anterior inferior aspect of vertebral body
- Classic imaging appearance: Height of triangular fragment is typically equal to or greater than its width
  - Height of fragment from "hyperextension dislocation injury" much less than width
- Other key facts
- Two types of teardrop fractures
  - Extension teardrop fracture
    - Mechanism is hyperextension
    - Anterior longitudinal ligament avulses anterior inferior aspect of vertebral body
    - Usually occurs at C2
    - May occur in lower cervical spine, especially in young patients
    - Usually considered a stable injury since only anterior column is involved
    - Patients are neurologically intact
  - Flexion teardrop fracture
    - Mechanism is hyperflexion with fracture-dislocation injury
    - Corner of lower vertebra impacts anterior inferior margin of upper vertebra and sheers off anterior inferior corner of vertebra
    - Usually occurs in lower cervical spine
    - Unstable injury since all three columns are involved
    - Devastating injury with complete quadriplegia and loss of pain, temperature and touch sensations
    - Flexion teardrop is a specific variation of the "burst fracture"

Teardrop Fractures

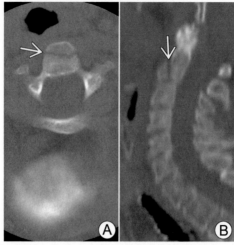

(A) Extension teardrop fracture at C2 is shown as anterior fracture line on axial image. (B) Sagittal reformation shows the characteristic triangular fragment from anterior inferior corner of vertebra. There is slight retrolisthesis of C2 on C3. There is no widening between the posterior elements of C2-3.

Imaging Findings

General Features

- Best imaging clue: Triangular fragment from anterior inferior corner of vertebral body
- Anatomy
  - Extension teardrop
    - Ligaments and disc are intact
  - Flexion teardrop
    - All ligaments and the disc are torn: Supraspinous, interspinous, ligamentum flavum, capsular ligaments, posterior longitudinal ligament (PLL), and anterior longitudinal ligament (ALL)

CT Findings

- Triangular fragment seen on sagittal reformations
- Soft tissue swelling of prevertebral soft tissues almost always occurs
- Other extension teardrop findings
  - Remainder of vertebral body and posterior elements are intact
  - Facet joints maintain normal apposition
- Other flexion teardrop findings
  - Other fractures of vertebral body as in burst fracture
  - Fractured vertebral body may be displaced posteriorly
  - Subluxation of facets
    - When subluxed, facet joint will appear widened posteriorly
  - Acute kyphosis at site of injury
  - Widening of interspinous and interlaminar distances

MR Findings

- Ligamentous damage and severe cord damage

Plain Film Findings

- Similar as findings above at CT

Teardrop Fractures

Imaging Recommendations
- Imaging of cervical spine trauma is best done with CT for assessment of fractures and alignment
- Neurological signs necessitate MR

Differential Diagnosis
- None relevant to this case

Pathology
- Stability may be assessed by "three column concept"
  - Anterior column: ALL plus anterior 2/3 of disc
  - Middle column: PLL plus posterior 1/3 of disc
  - Posterior column: All ligaments and bony structures posterior to PLL
  - Rule: Injury to two columns implies spinal instability

Clinical Issues
Presentation
- Extension teardrop
  - Pain
  - Muscle spasm
- Flexion teardrop
  - Anterior cervical cord syndrome including complete quadriplegia and loss of pain, temperature and touch sensations
  - Position, motion and vibration sensations are intact
Treatment
- With flexion teardrop fracture
  - Surgical decompression and fusion both anteriorly and posteriorly
- With extension teardrop fracture
  - Traction followed by collar
Prognosis
- Complete neurological findings do not improve

Selected References
1. Korres DS et al: The "tear drop" (or avulsed) fracture of the anterior inferior angle of the axis. Eur Spine J. 3:151-4, 1994
2. Cybulski GR et al: Complications in three-column spine injuries requiring anterior-posterior stabilization. Spine. 17:253-6, 1992
3. Torg JS, et al: The axial load teardrop fracture. A biomechanical, clinical and roentgenographic analysis. Am J Sports Med. 19:355-64, 1991

Cervical Burst Fracture

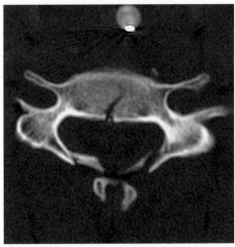

Axial CT image shows a fracture extending through the posterior cortex of the vertebral body. There are also fractures of the posterior elements.

Key Facts
- Definition: Comminution of the vertebral body due to axial loading resulting in the disk being driven into the vertebral body; usually fractures of the posterior elements also occur
- Classic imaging appearance: Fragment of bone from the posterior superior margin of the vertebra is displaced posteriorly into the spinal canal
- Other key facts
  - Spinal cord injury is frequent
  - Burst fractures are unstable injuries
  - The degree on comminution and orientation of fracture planes may vary
  - In the spine burst fracture may occur predominately on one side of the vertebral body

Imaging Findings
General Features
- Best imaging clue: Posterior herniation of vertebral body fragment
CT Findings
- Traditional burst fracture
  - One or more fragments may herniate posteriorly
  - Fracture of body is communited
  - The degree of compression of the vertebral body is variable, from severe to minimal
  - A sagittally oriented fracture through the inferior portion of the vertebral body is very frequent (90%), best appreciated on coronal reformations
  - Posterior elements are fractured very frequently (80+%)
- Lower cervical spine "teardrop fracture"
  - Specific form of burst fracture resulting from compression and flexion
  - Triangular piece of bone is noted at inferior anterior portion of vertebra

Cervical Burst Fracture

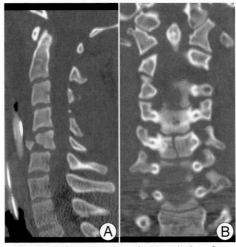

(A) Sagittal reformation in this patient shows the triangular bone fragment from the anterior inferior aspect of the vertebra, characteristic of the "teardrop" variation of the burst fracture. (B) Coronal reformation shows the sagittally oriented fracture through the C5 vertebral body.

- o Retrolisthesis of the vertebral body above the injury varies from minimal to significant posterior subluxation or dislocation
- o Posterior ligamentous injury with widening between posterior elements may occur
- o Disruption and widening of the facet joints may occur
- o A sagittally oriented fracture through the vertebral body is frequently seen, as in the traditional burst fracture

MR Findings
- The spinal cord, nerve roots, and injuries to these soft tissue structures are best demonstrated with MR

Plain Radiographic Findings
- Absence of all or a part of the posterior cortical line of the vertebral body due to the displacement of posterior fragment
- Minimal to severe compression of the vertebral body
- Posterior element fractures may be seen on oblique views
- Sagittal fracture though the vertebral body may be seen on the AP view

Imaging Recommendations
- CT is the modality of choice for screening or evaluating the cervical spine after significant trauma
- Technical parameters include image thickness and spacing of 2.5 mm, table speed of 3.75 mm/sec, and detector configuration of 4 x 1.25 mm

Differential Diagnosis
Compression Fracture
- Compression fractures involve axial loss of height of vertebral body

- In contrast to burst fractures, there is no fragmentation or posterior herniation of a vertebral body fragment & no fracture of posterior elements
- It may not be possible to differentiate mild burst from compression fracture with plain films

<u>Hyperextension Teardrop Fracture</u>
- Generally occurs at C2 or C3 due to avulsion of a triangular fragment from the anterior inferior corner of the vertebral body

Pathology
- None relevant to this case

Clinical Issues
<u>Presentation</u>
- Spinal cord injury including quadriplegia is very frequent

<u>Treatment</u>
- Surgery is usually necessary to stabilize the spine
- Outcome appears to be less favorable with halo-vest conservative treatment

Selected References
1. Koivikko MP et al: Conservative and operative treatment in cervical burst fractures. Arch Orthop Trauma Surg. 120:448-51, 2000
2. Torg JS et al: The axial load teardrop fracture. A biomechanical, clinical and roentgenographic analysis. Am J Sports Med. 19:355-64, 1991
3. Daffner RH et al: The posterior vertebral line: Importance in the detection of burst fractures. AJR Am J Roentgenol. 148:93, 1987

Traumatic Iso. Articular Pillar

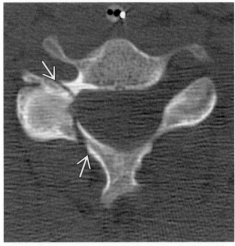

Traumatic isolation of the articular pillar (TIAP) involves ipsilateral fractures of the pedicle and lamina, which isolate the articular pillar from the remainder of the vertebra (arrows).

Key Facts
- Synonym(s): Fracture separation of the articular pillar
- Definition: Free floating articular pillar resulting from ipsilateral fractures of the pedicle and lamina, which attach the articular pillar to the remainder of the vertebra
- Classic imaging appearance
  - Fractures of pedicle and lamina allow the pillar to rotate
  - If the rotation occurs, this is easily seen on plain film lateral view or sagittal or coronal reformations from CT
- Other key facts
  - Type I injury involves minimal displacement of the articular pillar
  - Type II injury involves more displacement of the pillar and anterior translation of the vertebral body
  - Type III injury involves the findings in type II plus narrowing of an adjacent disc space
  - Type IV injury involves additional fracture of the pillar or subluxation or dislocation of the contralateral pillar

Imaging Findings
Plain Film Findings
- If rotation of the pillar occurs, this is pathognomonic of the TIAP and is seen on lateral view
- Oblique views may show the pedicle or lamina fractures
CT Findings
- Pedicle and lamina fractures are well seen on axial images
- Rotation may be in the sagittal or coronal plane and, if present, will be seen on the CT reformatted images

Differential Diagnosis
- None relevant to this case

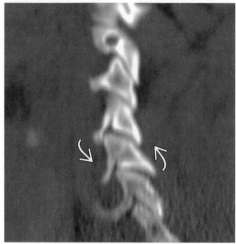

The articular pillar at C5 has rotated in the sagittal plain (arrows). The facet joint surfaces at the inferior margin of the articular pillar are no longer nearly parallel as the facets are at other levels.

Pathology

- Ipsilateral fractures of the pedicle and lamina are common to all types of injury
- Types of injury
  - Type I: Minimal displacement of the articular pillar
  - Type II: Displacement of the pillar and anterior translation of the vertebral body
  - Type III: Findings in type II plus narrowing of an adjacent disc space
  - Type IV: Additional fracture of the pillar or subluxation or dislocation of the contralateral pillar

Clinical Issues

Presentation

- Trauma with flexion while bending to the side
- 40-60% of patients with TIAP have neurological deficit
- Vertebral artery may be injured due to extension of fracture to transverse foramen

Selected References
1. Rhea JT: Rotational injuries of the cervical spine. Emergency Radiology 7:149-59, 2000
2. Shanmuganathan K, et al: Traumatic isolation of the cervical articular mass: Imaging observations in 21 patients. AJR Am J Roentgenol 166:897-902, 1996
3. Argenson C, et al: Traumatic rotatory displacement of the lower cervical spine. Spine 13:767-73, 1988

Hyperflexion Injury

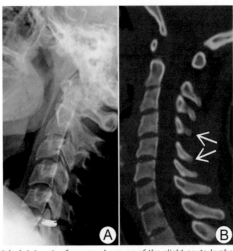

(A) Mild whiplash injury is of concern because of the slight acute kyphosis noted on the lateral plain film at C4-5 and minimal anterior subluxation of C4 on C5. (B) Sagittal reformation from CT shows findings seen on plain film plus widening of the interspinous distance (arrows). No fracture was present.

Key Facts
- Synonyms
  - Hyperflexion sprain or anterior subluxation injury
  - Whiplash could be considered a mild form of cervical sprain
- Definition: Injury of variable extent through the posterior and middle columns usually without fracture
- Classic imaging appearance: Acute kyphosis and widening of interspinous or interlaminar distance
- Mechanism
  - Whiplash: Abrupt flexion followed by extension as from deceleration in a low speed motor vehicle accident
  - Hyperflexion sprain: Distraction and flexion

Imaging Findings
General Features
- Straightening of the spine
- Angular kyphosis on lateral view
- Widening of the posterior elements, specifically the interspinous and interlaminar distances
- With severe injuries the disc and all ligaments except the anterior longitudinal ligament may be torn
Best Imaging Clue
- Acute kyphosis with or without slight anterolisthesis
CT Findings
- Angular kyphosis
- Widened interspinous and interlaminar distances
- Possible anterolisthesis of 1-3 mm
- Subluxation of articular pillars with slight widening at posterior aspect of facet joint

Hyperflexion Injury

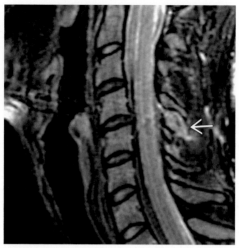

Sagittal MR scan indicates injury to interspinous ligament as seen by increased signal in this location (arrow).

<u>MR Findings</u>
- Ligamentous damage is well seen

<u>Plain Film Findings</u>
- Accentuation of abnormalities in flexion on lateral view
  - Acutely pain may prevent effective flexion with muscle spasm

<u>Imaging Recommendations</u>
- Cervical spine CT is indicated in initial assessment of trauma
- Alignment abnormality without fracture would be an indication for further assessment with MR
- Neurological signs or persistent pain would be an indication for MR

Differential Diagnosis

<u>Muscle Spasm</u>
- Smooth kyphotic curvature rather than angular kyphosis noted in spasm

<u>Flexion Teardrop Fracture</u>
- Fractures of vertebral body are not present in hyperflexion sprain

Pathology

<u>General</u>
- Ligamentous injuries include those of the posterior column and middle column
  - Posterior: Supraspinous, interspinous, ligamentum flavum, capsular ligaments
  - Middle: Posterior longitudinal ligament, posterior portion of disc

Clinical Issues

<u>Presentation</u>
- Pain and muscle spasm

<u>Treatment</u>
- Posterior fusion

Hyperflexion Injury

Prognosis
- Delayed instability and pain is noted in 30-50% of patients
- Vertebral and basilar artery dissection has been noted in patients with whiplash injury and other minor trauma

Selected References
1. Chung YS et al: Vertebrobasilar dissection: A possible role of whiplash injury in pathogenesis. Neurol Res. 24:129-38, 2002
2. Brady WJ et al: ED use of flexion-extension cervical spine radiography in the evaluation of blunt trauma. Am J Emerg Med. 17:504-8, 1999
3. Laporte C, et al: Severe hyperflexion sprains of the lower cervical spine in adults. Clin Orthop. 363:126-34, 1999

Articular Pillar Fracture

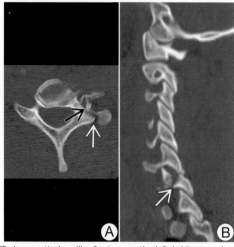

(A) Axial CT shows articular pillar fracture on the left (white arrow). The fracture extends into transverse foramen (black arrow). (B) The vertically oriented fracture (arrow) is seen best on the sagittal CT reformation. There is anterior subluxation of the pillar above the fracture, which is perched at the fracture edge.

Key Facts
- Synonym(s): Articular mass fracture (excluding C1 and C2 – see Hangman's fracture)
- Definition: Fracture of articular pillar
- Classic imaging appearance: Lucency through the articular pillar
- Other key facts
  - Unilateral fractures generally occur with some axial loading, extension and rotation; may also occur with flexion and rotation
  - Pillar fractures occur in about 20% of patients with cervical spine fractures
  - Occur frequently with facet dislocation when a corner of the pillar is sheared off – look for associated fractures
  - Radiculopathy is associated with pillar fracture
  - Pillar fractures may not be visible on plain films
  - Transverse process attaches to articular pillars
    - Fracture may extend to transverse foramen with possible injury to vertebral artery

Imaging Findings
General Features
- Best imaging clue: Lucency through articular pillar
- Other generic features: Fracture may be horizontal, vertical or oblique in orientation depending on the combination of forces at the time of injury
- Anatomy
  - Articular pillars are attached anteriorly to the vertebral body by the pedicle and posteriorly to the spinous process by the lamina
  - The joint surfaces between the articular pillars are called the articular facets and form the facet joints
    - Superior facet is the superior surface of the pillar
    - Inferior facet is the inferior surface of the pillar

Articular Pillar Fracture

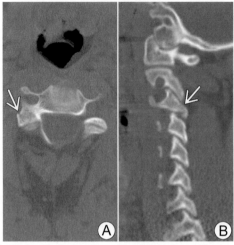

(A) C3 right articular pillar fracture (arrow) is subtle on the axial image. (B) Sagittal reformation shows compression of the posterior portion of the right articular pillar (arrow).

- o Rotation of the cervical spine occurs at the facet joints
  - Maximum rotation possible normally is about 90 degrees
  - Half of maximum rotation occurs at C1-2
  - The other half of maximum rotation occurs throughout the remainder of the facet joints

CT Findings
- Lucency through the articular pillar, which may or may not involve the facet surface
- Loss of height of part of the pillar may occur
- Horizontal fracture may be missed on single slice CT because resolution is insufficient and fracture is in the axial plane
- Reformations in the sagittal and coronal plane show the fracture to best advantage, especially with multi-slice scanners

Other Modality Findings
- Plain Film Findings
  - o AP view
    - Lateral most bony structure is the lateral edge of the articular pillars, which usually aligns in a smoothly undulating curve and which demonstrates cortical interruption with fracture
  - o Lateral view
    - Pillars are quadrilateral shapes projecting just behind the vertebral body, which may show lucency of fracture
  - o Oblique views
    - Pillars are not well seen because one side superimposes with the vertebral body and the other side superimposes with the lamina and spinous process
  - o Pillar views
    - The x-ray beam goes parallel to the facet joints in this AP view

- Usually two views need to be obtained with the mandible rotated first to one side, then the other side
- Lucency of fracture will be evident, especially if fracture in horizontal plane

Imaging Recommendations
- CT should be used to screen for fracture
- If plain films are done, any suspicious lucency should lead to CT

Differential Diagnosis
Cervical Spine Spondylolysis
- Cortical cleft between superior and inferior articular facets
- Equivalent lesion to the pars defect in the lumbar spine
- Associated dysplastic changes suggest this is congenital
- Lesion is well marginated with smooth edges

TIAP
- Traumatic isolation of the articular pillar (also called fracture separation of the articular pillar) occurs when the ipsilateral pedicle and lamina are fractured, thus isolating the pillar from the remainder of the vertebra
- A pillar fracture may occur from extension into the pillar of the pedicle or laminar fracture

Pathology
- None relevant to this case

Clinical Issues
Presentation
- Radiculopathy may be seen with isolated pillar fracture
- Muscle weakness
- Hypoesthesia
- Association with other fractures or dislocation may present with cord injury

Treatment
- Orthopedically applied appliance (orthosis) may be sufficient to allow healing
- More severe associated injuries may require surgical fusion, depending on the injury

Prognosis
- Isolated articular pillar fracture may heal in 3-4 months allowing resumption of activities
- Severe associated injuries may result in permanent cord damage

Selected References
1. Gleizes V et al: Combined injuries in the upper cervical spine: clinical and epidemiological data over a 14-year period. Eur Spine J. 9:386-92, 2000
2. Forsberg DA et al: Cervical spondylolysis; imaging findings in 12 patients. AJR 154:751-5, 1990
3. Yetkin Z et al: Uncovertebral and facet joint dislocations in cervical articular pillar fractures: CT evaluation. AJNR 6:633-7, 1985

Hyperextension Sprain

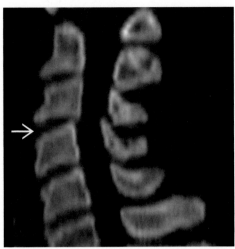

The findings of hyperextension sprain may be subtle. Sagittal reformation in the midline is needed to detect this injury at CT. There is widening of the disc space anteriorly at C3-4 (arrow). This is consistent with a hyperextension mechanism of injury.

Key Facts
- Synonym: Hyperextension dislocation
- Definition: Hyperextension force disrupts anterior longitudinal ligament and the anterior portion of the disc
- Classic imaging appearance on plain films or CT
  - Widening of the anterior aspect of the disc, usually in the lower cervical spine
  - Widening of the anterior aspect of the facet joints at the injured level
- Other key facts
  - Small linear fracture fragment may be pulled off the inferior end plate of the vertebra at the level of injury by fibers of the annulus of the disc
    - This fracture is longer than it is tall in contrast to triangular fragment seen in extension or flexion teardrop fractures
  - Upper vertebra displaces posteriorly
    - Impacts cord and may cause acute central spinal cord syndrome
    - Strips posterior longitudinal ligament off the lower vertebral body
  - Dislocation at time of injury reduces spontaneously
  - Lateral plain film may appear normal after this injury or the finding may be subtle
  - Sprain or sprain more frequent in younger patients, dislocation more frequent in older with degenerative changes

Imaging Findings
General Features
- Best imaging clue: Disproportionate widening between anterior aspect of vertebral bodies on lateral plain film

Hyperextension Sprain

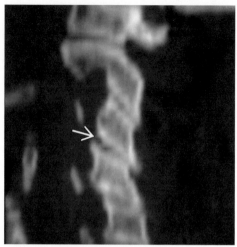

Sagittal reformation through articular masses of same patient. This image shows widening anteriorly at the facet joint of C3-4 (arrow).

CT Findings
- Soft tissue swelling
- Avulsion fracture from anterior aspect of inferior end plate will occur in about 2/3 of patients with this injury
- End plates of adjacent vertebrae widened anteriorly
- Facet joints widened anteriorly at level of injury
- Hyperextension may compress and fracture posterior elements

Imaging Recommendations
- Obtain MRI if patient has neurological findings

Differential Diagnosis

Extension Teardrop Fracture
- Extension results in avulsion on the anterior inferior corner of the vertebral body as a triangular shaped fragment

Hyperextension Fracture-Dislocation
- Severe form of hyperextension strain with vertebral displacement and posterior fractures

Pathology

General
- Cord contusion with edema and variable hemorrhagic necrosis

Clinical Issues

Presentation
- Central cord syndrome includes
  - Upper greater than lower extremity motor impairment
  - Variable sensory loss below level of injury
  - Variable loss of bowel, bladder, and sexual function

Treatment
- Surgery indicated if no neurological improvement or instability
  - Decompression may be indicated

- ○ Posterior and anterior plating with vertebral body fusion may be needed
- Steroids given in the acute setting
- Majority of patients are treated non-operatively
- Rehabilitation includes physical therapy

Prognosis
- Outcome is variable depending largely on age, with < 50 year olds having better prognosis; some recover completely, others may have permanent quadriplegia
- Recovery tends to begin in lower extremities, progressing to bladder and upper extremities

Selected References
1. Finnoff JT et al: Central cord syndrome in a football player with congenital spinal stenosis. Am J Sports Med 32:516-21, 2004
2. Gebhard JS et al: Soft tissue injuries of the cervical spine. Orthop Rev. Suppl:9-17, 1994
3. Gilula CE et al: The widened disk space: A sign of cervical hyperextension injury. Radiology. 141:639-44, 1981

PocketRadiologist®
ER-Trauma
Top 100 Diagnoses

THORACIC INJURY

Flail Chest

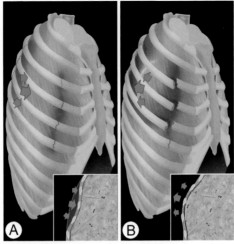

Flail chest. Multiple adjacent ribs are fractured in two or more places permitting a segment of chest to move independently with respiration. (A) Paradoxical motion is shown at inspiration in which the segment is sucked in rather than expanding to inflate right lung. (B) At expiration the segment is pushed out.

Key Facts
- Definition: Blunt trauma produces an incompetent segment of chest wall with paradoxical motion which impairs ventilation
- Classic imaging appearance
  - 5 or more adjacent ribs fractures in a row
  - 3 or more adjacent ribs are fractured in two or more places
  - Contusion of underlying lung
- Other key facts
  - Life threatening condition
  - Diagnosis is a combination of
    - Radiological findings of multiple rib fractures and lung injury
    - Clinical observation of paradoxical chest wall motion
    - Observation of physiological impairment of ventilation

Imaging Findings
Chest Films
- Multiple rib fractures; all fractures may not be seen on chest films
- Lung opacities may not be apparent on chest films
- Hemothorax
- Pneumothorax
- Subcutaneous emphysema
- Decreased size of involved hemithorax

CT Findings
- Multiple rib fractures
  - 5 or more adjacent ribs fractures in a row
  - 3 or more adjacent ribs are fractured in two or more places
- Underlying lung contusion
- Hemothorax
- Pneumothorax
- Decreased size of involved hemithorax

Flail Chest

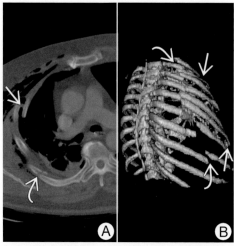

Right flail chest. (A) Axial bone window CT scan shows anterior (arrow) and posterior (curved arrows) rib fractures. Right chest is smaller than left with a right hemothorax and atelectasis. (B) 3D CT showing two vertical rows of anterior (arrows) and posterior (curved arrows) rib fractures margining flail segment.

- Subcutaneous emphysema

Imaging Recommendations
- Chest CT with IV contrast material
- View lung, soft tissue and bone windows of CT scan
- 3D reformation of chest wall may be helpful

Differential Diagnosis
Multiple Rib Fractures Without Flail Chest
- No free segment of chest wall with paradoxical or reverse motion

Pathology
General
- General Path Comments
  - Multiple rib fractures
  - Fractures permit a free-floating segment of chest wall
  - 3 factors impair ventilation
    - Interruption of normal negative pressure needed to effect inflation of ipsilateral lung due to paradoxical chest wall motion
    - Pulmonary contusion of underlying lung
    - Pain from multiple fractures results in splinting with subsequent hypoventilation
  - Outcome related to extent of contusion and size of flail segment
- Etiology
  - Blunt trauma or crushing injury to chest from motor vehicle collisions, falls and assaults
  - Flail chest indicates high kinetic energy trauma
  - In older, osteoporotic individuals may occur with less severe trauma
  - Flail chest less common in children due to a more compliant chest wall
- Epidemiology

o American College of Surgeons has estimated approximately 1-2 cases per month for each level one trauma center

Clinical Issues
Presentation
- Blunt trauma patients with paradoxical or reverse motion of the chest wall while spontaneously breathing
- This clinical finding will disappear with positive pressure ventilation which may mask the presence of flail chest
- The degree of respiratory deficiency is related to the extent of underlying lung injury

Treatment
- Complete pain relief with narcotic and thoracic epidurals to aid patient tolerance of ventilation
- Aggressive pulmonary toilet
- Mechanical ventilation reserved for those patients who do not respond to conservative measures
- Internal fixation of rib fractures many be indicated in some patients to improve recovery by reducing ventilator time and ventilator associated complications

Prognosis
- Long term disability in some patients, including persistent chest wall pain, deformity and dyspnea on exertion
- Most patients do well and return to normal function after 6-12 months

Selected References
1. Gurney JW: ABC's of blunt chest trauma. Thoracic Imaging. Society of Thoracic Radiology Syllabus 349-52, 1996
2. Freedland M et al: JS. The management of flail chest injury: factors affecting outcome. J Trauma 30:1460-9, 1990
3. Ciraulo DL et al: Flail chest as a marker for significant injuries. J Am Coll Surg 178:466-70, 1994

Sternal Fracture

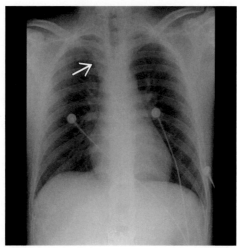

Sternal Fracture. PA chest film shows widening (arrow) of the upper right mediastinum due to the presence of mediastinal hematoma. The aortic arch is normal. No fracture is seen on the chest film.

Key Facts
- Synonym: Manubrial Fracture
- Classic imaging appearance
  - Demonstration of a simple or displaced sternal fracture
- Other key facts
  - Often resulting from an anterior blow to the sternum in a motor vehicle collision
  - Always consider possible associated cardiac or great vessel injury

Imaging Findings
General Findings
- Sternal fracture
- Mediastinal hematoma
- Signs of cardiac or great vessel injury

Chest Film Findings
- Sternal fractures not usually visible on frontal chest films
- Retrosternal hematoma associated with sternal fractures may produce mediastinal widening on frontal chest films
- Mediastinal widening occurring with sternal fractures may be confused with signs of aortic injury
- On plain films, sternal fractures best seen on a lateral view or other special view of the sternum

CT Findings
- CT will show nearly all sternal fractures
- Coronal and sagittal CT reformations will best show horizontal fractures of the sternum
- Mediastinal hematoma associated with sternal fractures is seen in the retrosternal-anterior mediastinum, anterior to the aorta and other great vessels

Sternal Fracture

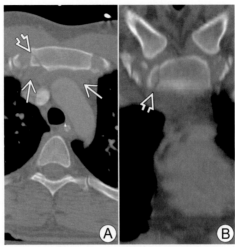

Sternal Fracture. (A) Axial CT scan, bone window. (Open arrow) indicates a fracture of manubrial segment of right sternum. (Arrows) indicate anterior (retrosternal) mediastinal hematoma anterior to aorta and great vessels, aorta appears normal. (B) Coronal CT reformation showing fracture line (open arrow).

- Common sign of associated cardiac injury at CT is presence of hemopericardium

Imaging Recommendations
- Lateral plain film of the sternum
- CT with coronal and sagittal reformations of the sternum
- CT examination should be performed with IV contrast material to assist in diagnosis of possible cardiac or great vessel injury

Differential Diagnosis
Sternoclavicular Dislocation
Anterior Rib Fracture
Costochondral Fracture
Cardiac or Great Vessel Injury

Pathology
General
- General Path Comments
  - Depressed sternal body fractures may be associated with myocardial injuries, including myocardial laceration
  - Manubrial fractures may be associated with injuries of aorta and brachiocephalic blood vessels (great vessels)
  - 40% of sternal fractures associated with compression fractures of upper thoracic spine
  - Less commonly sternal fractures are associated with cervical and lumbar spine fractures
- Etiology-Pathogenesis
  - Direct anterior blow to the sternum
  - In motor vehicle collisions blow may be caused by steering wheel, shoulder belt or airbag

Sternal Fracture

- o Sternal fractures may result from cardiac resuscitation
- o Spontaneous sternal fractures may be seen in osteoporotic, elderly persons with a thoracic kyphosis
- Epidemiology
- o Seen in approximately 3% of motor vehicle collisions

Gross Pathologic, Surgical Features

- Sternal fractures are usually transverse involving the sternal body
- Fractures may be non-displaced or displaced; when displaced the lower fragment is usually displaced posteriorly
- Retrosternal-anterior mediastinal hematoma see with most fractures
- Retrosternal hematoma confined by the parietal pleura

Clinical Issues

Presentation

- Sternal pain and tenderness
- Pain associated with spontaneous sternal fractures in osteoporotic patients may be confused with acute myocardial ischemia

Treatment

- Non-displaced, simple fractures are treated conservatively
- Depressed fractures may require open reduction and fixation
- Since depressed fractures have a higher association with cardiac injury, echocardiography, CT or other cardiac tests are recommended to rule out pericardial effusion or other signs of myocardial injury

Prognosis

- Prognosis is good with simple sternal fractures having no signs of cardiac or great vessel injury
- Non-union of sternal fractures has been observed

Selected References
1. Stern EJ et al: The thoracic cage. In Rogers LF, editor, Radiology of Skeletal Trauma, 3rd edition, Churchill Livingstone, New York, 2002
2. Huggett JM et al: CT findings of sternal fracture. Injury. 29;623, 1998
3. Hills MW et al: Sternal fractures: Associated injuries and management. J. Trauma. 35:55-60. 1993

Scapular Fracture

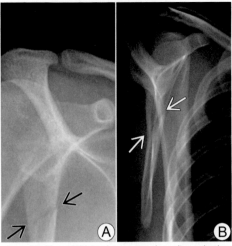

Scapular Fracture. (A) AP and (B) lateral, transscapular radiographs through the right shoulder demonstrate the oblique fracture of the scapular body (arrows).

Key Facts
- Synonym: Broken shoulder blade
- Definition: Disruption of the scapular bone
- Classic imaging appearance: Lucent line with irregular margins at the site of fracture
- Classification
  - Body or spine fracture (most common)
  - Acromion fracture
  - Neck fracture
  - Glenoid fracture
  - Coracoid fracture

Imaging Findings
General Features
- Best imaging clue: Identification of the fracture lucency
- Anatomy
  - Bony connection between the upper arm and the thorax
  - Scapular glenoid articulates with the humeral head
  - Scapular acromion and coracoid processes connect the scapula to the clavicle
  - Scapula is covered by muscle layers, responsible for the smooth movement
Radiography Findings
- AP shoulder
  - Shows fracture lucencies through different aspects of the scapula
- Lateral scapular: Necessary for two-plane evaluation of the scapula
- Lateral axillary
  - Transverse lucent line through the coracoid process
  - Delineates associated shoulder dislocations
  - Acromial fractures may be seen as irregularity of the acromial margin rather than a lucent fracture line

Scapular Fracture

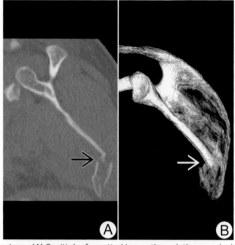

Scapular Fracture. (A) Sagittal reformatted image through the scapula demonstrates comminuted fracture of the scapular body (arrow). (B) 3D reformatted CT image in the same patient illustrates the dimensions of the comminuted scapular fracture (arrow).

CT Findings
- NECT: Glenoid and coracoid fracture assessment

MR Findings
- T1WI: Dark signal intensity of the fracture line
- T2WI
  - High signal intensity of the fracture line
  - High signal intensity within the injured soft tissue such as ligaments, glenoid labrum and joint effusion
- Inversion recovery sequences: Ideal for evaluation of edema, which is high signal

Imaging Recommendations
- AP shoulder is essential to rule out articular involvement
- CT scans of the abdomen and chest are occasionally indicated to assess possible associated injuries

Differential Diagnosis
Os Acromiale
- Secondary ossification center of acromion
- Best seen on the axillary view
- Comprises the entire anterior end of the acromion
- Usually fuses by age 24
- Differentiation from fracture made by location and also corticated margins

Pathology
General
- Etiology-Pathogenesis
  - Body or spine fractures: Severe direct force, as in a fall or motor vehicle accident

Scapular Fracture

- o Acromion fracture: Downward force to the shoulder
  - ▪ Superiorly displaced fractures: As the result of a superior dislocation of the shoulder
- o Neck fracture: Direct anterior or posterior force to the shoulder
- o Glenoid fracture: Fall onto a flexed elbow
  - ▪ Stellate fracture of the glenoid: Direct lateral force
- o Coracoid fracture: Usually result from 1 of 2 mechanisms
  - ▪ Direct force to the superior point of the shoulder or the humeral head in an anterior shoulder dislocation
  - ▪ Avulsion fracture from abrupt contractions of the coracoacromial muscle, short head of the biceps, or coracohumeral muscle
- Epidemiology
  - o More common among men because of their increased incidence of significant blunt trauma
  - o Predominantly in 20-40 years of age, because of the increased occurrence of significant blunt trauma in this population
  - o Scapular fractures occur in less than 1% of all fractures

Clinical Issues

Presentation
- Tenderness, edema, and ecchymosis over the affected area
- Limited range of motion, flattened shoulder, painful breathing
- Up to 80% of scapular fractures associated with injuries to the chest wall, lungs, and shoulder

Natural History
- The most common complication of an isolated scapular fracture is posttraumatic arthritis or bursitis

Treatment
- Body of scapula
  - o Immobilization with sling
  - o Ice packs and pain medications for pain relief
  - o Physical therapy as early as one week after the injury
- Neck or glenoid involvement in scapular fracture: Surgical reduction

Prognosis
- If no significant associated injury exists, the prognosis of scapular body fracture is excellent
- Fractures of the scapular neck and scapular glenoid more likely to have complications such as impaired strength and also range of motion, persistent pain and finally early arthritis

Selected References
1. Kopecky KK et al: CT diagnosis of fracture of the coracoid process of the scapula. Comput. Radiol. 8:325, 1984
2. Mc Gahan JP et al: Fractures of the scapula. J. Trauma. 20:880, 1980
3. Wilber MC et al: Fractures of the scapula. J. Bone Joint. Surg. [Am] 59:358, 1977

Sternoclavicular Dislocation

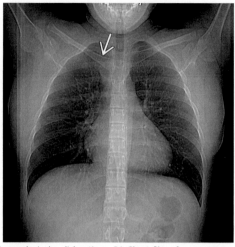

Posterior stermoclavicular dislocation. PA Chest film of a young woman who fell down a flight of stairs receiving a posterior blow to the right shoulder. The film shows asymmetry of the medial heads of the clavicles. The right medical clavicle (arrow) is positioned slightly lower than the left.

Key Facts
- Definition: Dislocation between the medial head of the clavicle and superiolateral margin of manubrium
  - Both anterior or posterior dislocation may occur
- Classic imaging appearance
  - Difficult to diagnose on conventional plain film radiographs, including special plain film projections of the sternoclavicular joint
  - Chest film may show the affected medial clavicle lying at a different level than the opposite side
  - With posterior dislocation there may be mediastinal widening due to mediastinal hematoma
  - Sternoclavicular dislocation best diagnosed by CT
- Other key facts
  - Diagnosis may be difficult to establish due to rarity of the condition and difficulty imaging the sternoclavicular joint on conventional radiographs

Imaging Findings
Plain Film Findings
- On frontal chest films, asymmetry of the clavicles, with or without mediastinal widening
CT Findings
- CT shows precise relationship between medical clavicles and manubrium
- Anterior and posterior dislocation clearly depicted by CT
- With posterior dislocation injuries of the great vessels, trachea and esophagus may also be identified
Imaging Recommendations
- CT with IV contrast is preferred imaging technique
- Both bone and soft tissue windows should be reviewed

Sternoclavicular Dislocation

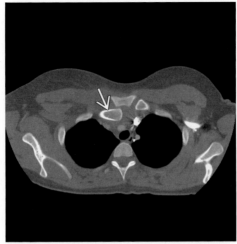

Posterior sternoclavicular dislocation. Bone window CT scan through the sternoclavicular joints shows posterior dislocation of the right medial clavicle (arrow). Compare with the left. Hemorrhage can be seen in the anterior mediastinum but no injury is identified of the trachea or blood vessels.

- Evaluate vascular structures for possible injury with posterior dislocation

Differential Diagnosis
Clavicle Fracture
Sternal Fracture

Pathology
General
- General Path Comments
  - Sternoclavicular dislocation disrupts the ligaments of the sternoclavicular joint
- Etiology-Pathogenesis
  - Anterior dislocations result from an anterior blow to the shoulder
    - Clavicle acts as a lever producing an anterior disruption of the sternoclavicular joint
  - Posterior dislocation usually results from a posterior blow to the shoulder that forces the medial clavicle posteriorly
  - Posterior dislocation may also result from a direct anterior blow to the medial clavicle
  - Posterior dislocations are more serious due to possible injury of the aorta, brachiocephalic blood vessels, trachea, esophagus or brachial plexus
- Epidemiology
  - Uncommon, representing 2-3% of shoulder girdle dislocations
  - Anterior dislocations more frequent than posterior dislocations
  - Most dislocations occur in young people less than 25 years
  - Sternoclavicular dislocations in the young may represent separations of the medial clavicle epiphysis

Sternoclavicular Dislocation

Clinical Issues

Presentation

- Pain in the affected sternoclavicular joint
- On physical examination tenderness over affected joint as well as a palpable or visible contour abnormality

Treatment

- Reduction of dislocation
- Management of any associated injuries of blood vessels, trachea or esophagus

Selected References
1. Lenchik L: The shoulder and humeral shaft. Radiology of Skeletal Trauma, 3rd edition. Churchill Livingstone, New York, 2002
2. Destouet JM et al: Computed tomography of the sternoclavicular joint and sternum. Radiology 138:123, 1981
3. Levinsohn EM et al: Computed tomography in the diagnosis of dislocations of the sternoclavicular joint. Clin. Orthop, 140:12, 1979

Occult Pneumothorax

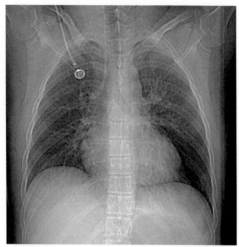

Bilateral occult pneumothoraces. AP chest film of a young multiple trauma patient does not show a definite pneumothorax. Slight increased lucency in the left lower chest and slightly better definition of the left heart border presumably result from the large left pneumothorax easily seen at CT.

Key Facts
- Definition
  - A pneumothorax is a condition in which air enters the pleural space
  - An occult pneumothorax is one which is not diagnosed on a plain chest film but readily seen by CT
- Classic imaging appearance
  - Unremarkable chest film; air in the pleural space at CT
- Other key facts
  - In trauma patients radiographed in the supine position, air in a pneumothorax floats anteriorly and may not be visible on a chest film
  - Such an occult pneumothorax is easily detected by CT
  - Increasing use of CT in trauma has increased the detection of occult pneumothoraces
  - In many reported trauma investigations, nearly half the pneumothoraces identified at CT were occult, not visible on the initial portable chest film
  - Both spontaneous (not cased by trauma) and traumatic pneumothoraces may be occult

Imaging Findings
General Features
Chest Films
- An occult pneumothorax is not readily seen on a supine chest film
- A pneumothorax not seen on a supine chest film may be seen on an upright chest film, especially one taken at expiration
- The signs of an occult pneumothorax on a supine chest film may include
  - A deep sulcus sign (very wide and deep ipsilateral costophrenic sulcus)

Occult Pneumothorax

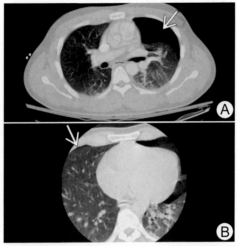

Bilateral occult pneumothoraces. (A) Lung window chest CT scan at level of pulmonary arteries shows a large left pneumothorax (arrow). (B) Coned-down CT scan at level of heart shows an additional small right pneumothorax (arrow).

CT Findings
- Lung window axial slices show air within the pleural space

Imaging Recommendations
- CT with IV contrast material is the most accurate imaging technique for the detection of thoracic injuries including occult pneumothoraces

Differential Diagnosis
- Pneumomediastinum
  - Air in the mediastinum which may reflect an injury of the tracheobronchial tree or esophagus

Pathology

General
- General Path Comments
  - Injury to the visceral pleura of the lung resulting in air accumulation within the pleural space
- Etiology-Pathogenesis
  - May be caused by blunt or penetrating trauma
  - May occur in trauma when the lung is punctured by a fractured rib
  - Spontaneous pneumothoraces are associated with the rupture of pulmonary blebs and bullae and with emphysema
  - Iatrogenic causes of pneumothorax include vascular line placement, lung biopsy, and mechanical ventilation

Grading Criteria
- Occult pneumothoraces have been graded as
  - (1) Miniscule (small)
  - (2) Anterior (moderate)
  - (3) Anterolateral (large)

Occult Pneumothorax

Clinical Issues

Presentation

- Dyspnea and ipsilateral chest pain
- Physical findings of pneumothoraces include tachypnea, hypoxia, cyanosis and hypotension
- Decreased ipsilateral breath sounds at auscultation

Natural History

- Untreated small and moderate-sized occult pneumothoraces resolve
- All pneumothoraces may increase in size with positive pressure ventilation

Treatment

- Conservative management for small and moderate-sized occult pneumothoraces
- Large and/or symptomatic occult pneumothoraces generally require treatment with tube thoracostomy and suction
- All pneumothoraces require tube thoracostomy and suction if a patient will under go positive pressure ventilation for general anesthesia or assisted ventilation

Prognosis

- Correctly diagnosed and treated pneumothoraces have a good prognosis

Selected References
1. Misthos P et al: A prospective analysis of occult pneumothorax, delayed pneumothorax and delayed hemothorax after minor blunt thoracic trauma. Eur J Cardiothorac Surg. 25(5):859-64, 2004
2. Hill SL et al: The occult pneumothorax: An increasing diagnostic entity in trauma. Am Surg 65:254-8, 1999
3. Wolfman NT et al: Validity of CT classification on management of occult pneumothorax: A prospective study. AJR 171:1317-20, 1998

Tension Pneumothorax

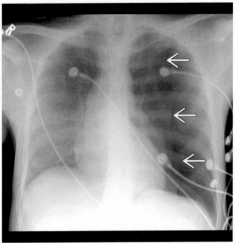

Tension pneumothorax. Frontal chest film reveals a large left pneumothorax (arrows) associated with mediastinal shift to the right (compare with image on next page), depression of the left hemidiaphragm and increased volume of the left hemithorax with splaying of the left ribs. Note tracheal deviation to the right.

Key Facts
- Definition: The accumulation of air under pressure in the pleural space
- Classic imaging appearance
  - A pneumothorax associated with shift of the mediastinum to the opposite side
- Other key facts
  - Life-threatening condition
  - Develops when injured lung tissue forms a one-way valve
    - Air enters pleural space and is prevented from escaping naturally
  - Condition rapidly progresses to respiratory insufficiency, cardiovascular collapse and ultimately death
  - Favorable outcome requires immediate diagnosis and treatment

Imaging Findings
Best Imaging Clue: Pneumothorax with Mediastinal Shift
- Chest Film Findings
  - Pneumothorax
  - Mediastinal shift with tracheal deviation to the opposite side
  - Depression of the ipsilateral hemidiaphragm
  - Increased volume of the ipsilateral hemithorax with splaying of the ipsilateral ribs
Imaging Recommendations
- Many clinicians believe that a tension pneumothorax, especially when severe, is a clinical diagnosis and needle aspiration should be performed immediately, with a chest film only after tube thoracostomy
- Chest radiography is diagnostic when performed and is especially helpful in the early stages of this condition
- Repeat chest film after treatment can document resolution of tension

Tension Pneumothorax

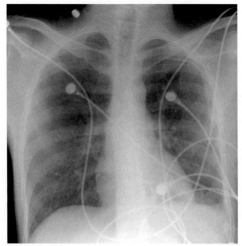

Tension pneumothorax: Frontal chest following treatment with needle aspiration and tube thoracostomy. Mediastinal shift, tracheal deviation, depression of left hemidiaphragm and splaying of left ribs have all resolved.

Differential Diagnosis
<u>Simple Pneumothorax</u>
- No shift of the mediastinum, depression of the ipsilateral hemidiaphragm nor splaying of the ipsilateral ribs

Pathology
<u>General</u>
- General Path Comments
  - o Injury to visceral pleura with a rapid one-way accumulation of air within the pleural space
  - o Intrapleural pressure increases causing
    - Collapse of ipsilateral lung with hypoxia
    - Compression of mediastinal structures with impingement of venous structures entering right atrium
  - o Venous return to heart is impaired resulting in severe hemodynamic instability associated with worsening hypoxia
- Etiology-Pathogenesis
  - o Any pneumothorax can become a tension pneumothorax
  - o Pneumothoraces may be spontaneous, traumatic or iatrogenic
  - o Common causes are
    - Blunt or penetrating trauma
    - Barotrauma associated with positive-pressure ventilation
    - Central venous catheter placement
    - Chest compression during cardiopulmonary resuscitation
    - Percutaneous lung biopsy
- Epidemiology
  - o Pneumothoraces occur in 15-40% of patients with non-penetrating trauma
  - o The overall incidence of tension pneumothorax is not known

Tension Pneumothorax

Clinical Issues

Presentation

- Early clinical findings
  - Chest pain, dyspnea, anxiety, tachypnea, tachycardia
  - Decreased breath sounds and hyper-resonance on affected side
- Late clinical findings
  - Deviation of the trachea away from the affected side
  - Hypotension
  - Cyanosis
  - Decreased level of consciousness

Treatment

- Life-threatening condition that demands urgent management
- Start 100% oxygen
- Immediate needle decompression of air from the pleural space
- Tube thoracostomy after needle decompression
- Follow-up radiograph for confirmation
- Monitor patient continuously for arterial oxygen saturation

Prognosis

- Early diagnosis and prompt treatment promote a good prognosis
- Overall patient prognosis related to presence of other injuries and other medical conditions

Selected References

1. Vinson ED: Improvised chest tube drain for decompression of an acute tension pneumothorax. Mil Med. 169(5):403-5, 2004
2. Friend KD: Prehospital recognition of tension pneumothorax. PreHosp Emerg Care. 1:75-77, 2000
3. Wiot JF: The radiologic manifestations of blunt chest trauma. JAMA. 231:500-503, 1975

Hemothorax

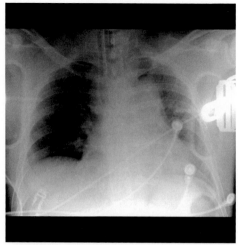

Hemothorax. Increased overall density in the left hemithorax represents a layered out hemothorax in this supine patient. The mediastinum is widened and the aortic arch shadow is increased in size and abnormal in contour in this patient with aortic trauma and mediastinal hematoma.

Key Facts
- Synonym(s): Hematothorax, Intrathoracic hemorrhage
- Definition: Accumulation of blood in the pleural space
- Classic imaging appearance
  - Pleural fluid in a trauma patient
  - Fluid measures high density (blood density) at CT
  - May be associated with a pneumothorax or other signs of chest trauma
- Other key facts
  - Trauma is most common cause of hemothorax
  - May result from blunt or penetrating trauma

Imaging Findings
General Features
- Best imaging clue
  - Fluid in pleural space of a trauma patient
Chest Film Findings
- Fluid in pleural space
  - On supine film fluid layers out producing an overall increased density in affected hemithorax
  - May require upright or decubitus plain films, or a CT scan to confirm a hemothorax
- Pneumothorax, rib fractures or other signs of chest trauma may be present
- With large/massive hemothorax may see collapse of ipsilateral lung and mediastinal shift
CT Findings
- Fluid in pleural space is blood density (> 40 HU)
- A fluid-fluid level may be seen representing sedimentation of red cells

Hemothorax

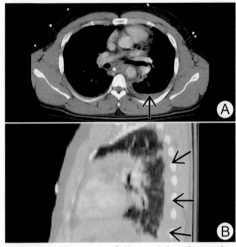

Hemothorax. (A) Axial CT scan at soft tissue window shows a layered-out left hemothorax (arrow). The fluid measured 45 HU at CT consistent with blood density. (B) Sagittal reformation through the left chest viewed with a lung window again shows the layered-out left hemothorax (arrows).

- Active bleeding into the pleural space may be recognized by extravasation of IV contrast material into the hemothorax
- CT may show lung laceration or other injury responsible for the hemothorax

Imaging Recommendations
- Plain film of the chest
  - Upright or decubitus films for small hemothorax
- Chest CT with IV contrast material
  - Perform sagittal and coronal CT reformations
  - Look for active bleeding

Differential Diagnosis
Traumatic Chylothorax
- Lymphatic fluid in the pleural space due to leakage of chyle from an injury of the thoracic duct or one its tributaries
- Diagnosis made by thoracentesis and pleural fluid analysis
Pleural Effusion
- Low density pleural fluid usually under 10 HU at CT
- Thoracentesis and pleural fluid analysis
Non-Traumatic Hemothorax
- Associated with thoracic surgery, pulmonary embolism with infarction, neoplasm, aortic dissection, thoracic aortic aneurysm or anticoagulation

Pathology
General
- General Path Comments
  - Blood enters pleural space from injuries to blood vessels of the chest wall, lung, mediastinum or diaphragm

Hemothorax

- Etiology-Pathogenesis
  - Blunt or penetrating trauma
  - With blunt trauma hemothorax usually associated with a chest wall or pulmonary injury such as a fractured rib or lung laceration
  - With penetrating trauma usually a result of a direct laceration of a blood vessel with the chest wall, lung or mediastinum
- Epidemiology
  - One of the most common manifestations of chest trauma
  - Chest injuries occur in approximately 60% of multiple trauma patients
    - Rough estimate of hemothorax would be about 300,000 cases per year in the US

Staging or Grading Criteria
- May be graded subjectively as small, medium, large or massive hemothorax
  - Large/massive may be associated with mediastinal shift and cardio-respiratory compromise

Clinical Issues

Presentation
- History and signs of chest trauma
- Chest pain, tachypnea and dyspnea
- Dullness to chest percussion on affected side
- Auscultation reveals decreased breath sounds on affected side
- If respiratory failure ensues patient will appear anxious, restless, stuporous and cyanotic

Natural History
- Bleeding may be self-limited and small
  - Mild hemothorax will resolve in 10 to 14 days
- Large hemothorax can interfere with breathing
  - Blood takes up space that lung would use for ventilation
- Hemothorax with active bleed can result in exsanguination
  - Pleural space of an adult can hold 4 or more liters
    - Sufficient space to permit exsanguinating hemorrhage (hemothorax) without external evidence of blood loss
- Empyema may result from bacterial contamination of a hemothorax

Treatment
- Evacuation by chest tube to evacuated blood and re-expand lung
  - Permits physician to monitor for persistent bleeding
  - Prevents organization of hemothorax which can progress to fibrothorax and subsequent lung entrapment
- Persistent hemothorax after chest tube placement and suction may due to bronchial injury, vascular injury or malfunctioning or malpositioned chest tube
- Thoracotomy may required to evacuated blood clots which cannot be removed by chest tube and to control active bleeding

Prognosis
- Good for small hemothorax

Selected References
1. Rusch VW et al: Chest wall, pleura, lung and mediastinum. Schwartz SI, ed. Principles of Surgery. 7th ed. New York, NY: McGraw-Hill, 1999
2. Parry GW et al: Management of Haemothorax. Ann R Coll Surg Engl 78:325-6, 1996
3. Richardson JD et al: Complex thoracic injuries. Surg Clin North Am 76:725-48, 1996

Lung Contusion

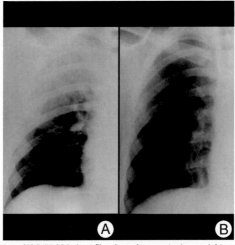

Lung contusion. (A) Initial PA chest film shows lung contusion as right upper lobe air-space opacity. (B) Repeat chest film three days later shows complete clearing.

Key Facts
- Definition: A bruise of the lung parenchyma due to blunt trauma
- Classic imaging appearance
  - Non-segmental, patchy, air-space opacities which do not recognize any anatomical boundaries
- Other key facts
  - Most common lung injury with blunt trauma
  - Contusion is differentiated from pulmonary aspiration by the distribution of air space opacities which is segmental with aspiration

Imaging Findings
General Features
- Best imaging clue
  - Non-segmental airspace opacities
- Other generic features
  - Opacities are peripheral and occur under the site of injury
  - Both coup and contra-coup contusions may be seen
  - Rib fractures often seen over coup sites
  - A thin margin of sparing may be noted at the pleural surface of contusions
  - 85% appear within the first 6 hours; 100% in 12-24 hours
  - Contusions start clearing in 2-4 days; complete resolution within 4-10 days
  - If new pulmonary opacities appear in trauma patients after 24 hours, consider aspiration or superimposed infection rather than contusion
  - Air bronchograms may be seen but more often blood clots in the bronchi opacify the airways
  - Contusions may occur independently or may be associated with pulmonary lacerations which may not become visible on radiographs until the contusion clear

Lung Contusion

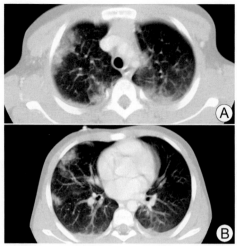

Lung contusion. (A, B) Lung window chest CT scans shows multiple patchy air-space opacities in both lungs in a non-segmental pattern typical for lung contusion.

Chest Films
- Non-segmental, patchy, ill-defined parenchymal opacities which may be multiple or solitary
- Large contusions well shown on plain films; small contusions may be overlooked

CT Findings
- Contusions more precisely shown with CT
- Also better shown are other injuries associated with contusion including rib fractures and lung lacerations

Imaging Recommendations
- Chest CT with IV contrast material; review images on lung, soft tissue and bone windows

Differential Diagnosis
Pulmonary Aspiration
- Although aspiration produces air-space consolidations in the lungs of trauma patients, the opacities are segmental in distribution and are usually restricted to the dependent portions of the lungs
- Contusion start to clear in 2-4 days and aspiration will not clear so quickly

Pathology
General
- General Path Comments
  - Combination of alveolar hemorrhage with interstitial hemorrhage and interstitial edema
  - In adults associated with overlying rib fractures
  - In children and young adults, the ribs are more pliable and may not fracture when contusion occurs
  - Hemorrhage, edema and inflammation of the affected lung result in decreased oxygenation and impaired ventilation
- Etiology-Pathogenesis

Lung Contusion

- o Blunt chest trauma
  - Blow to the chest produces a pressure wave which compresses the thoracic cavity, injuring the underlying lung
- o Penetrating chest trauma
  - Contusion may be seen outlining the bullet track of a lung gunshot wound, or outlining the laceration of a lung stab wound
- Epidemiology
  - o The most frequent lung injury with blunt trauma

Clinical Issues

Presentation
- Contusion may present with dyspnea, tachypnea, tachycardia and hemoptysis

Natural History
- Most lung contusions resolve without specific treatment within a week
- Massive lung contusion may lead to respiratory failure and adult respiratory distress syndrome

Treatment
- Conservative management with fluid replacement, aggressive pulmonary toilet, pain control and oxygen therapy
- No specific medical treatment for contusion

Prognosis
- Good for small and moderate-sized contusions
- Massive lung contusion has been associated with a 30% mortality rate

Selected References
1. Kuhlman JE et al: Radiographic and CT findings of blunt chest trauma: Aortic injuries and looking beyond the. Radiographics 18:1085-1106, 1998
2. Kollmorgen DR et al: Predictors of mortality in pulmonary contusion. Am J Surg 168:659, 1994
3. Wiot JF: The radiologic manifestations of blunt chest trauma. JAMA 231:500-3, 1975

Lung Laceration

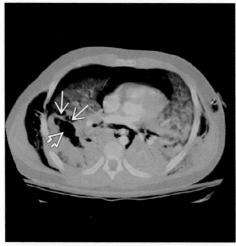

Lung lacerations: Lung window chest CT scan. Open arrow indicates a large right lung laceration. Arrows indicate two smaller lacerations. Extensive air-space opacities represent both contusion and aspiration (posteriorly). Pneumothoraces, pneumomediastinum and subcutaneous emphysema are also present.

Key Facts
- Synonyms: Pulmonary laceration, pulmonary hematoma, traumatic pneumatocele
- Definition: Traumatic disruption of the lung parenchyma
- Classic imaging appearance
  - A tear in the lung parenchyma containing air, fluid or an air-fluid level
- Other key facts
  - Lacerations may be caused by blunt or penetrating trauma
  - When a laceration fills with air, called a traumatic pneumatocele
  - When a laceration fills with blood, called a traumatic hematocele or pulmonary hematoma
  - When a laceration fills with both blood and air, called a traumatic hematopneumatocele
  - Initially a laceration is surrounded by contusion which usually resolves within the first week making the laceration visible or more apparent

Imaging Findings
General Features
- Lacerations becomes round in shape due to the inherent lung elasticity
- They may not display a classical round appearance for the first few days until surrounding contusion clears
- Usually 2-5 cm in diameter although may be as large as 10-15 cm
- May be solitary or multiple
- Many acute lung lacerations contain both air and blood and show an air-fluid level on plain films and CT
- Plain Chest Films

Lung Laceration

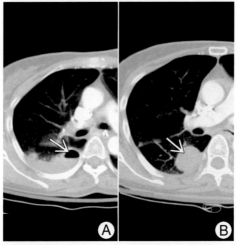

Lung laceration. (A) Initial CT scan shows a small lung laceration (arrow) with an air-fluid level (hematopneumatocele), surrounded by contusion and a small right hemothorax. (B) One week later the contusion and hemothorax have resolved and the air in the laceration has resorbed leaving a pulmonary hematoma (arrow).

- o Laceration are difficult to diagnose acutely on plain films as they are masked by surrounding contusion
- o Later they appear as a spherical soft tissue densities which could be confused with a malignant pulmonary nodules
- CT Findings
  - o Spherical or linear holes within the lung containing, air, fluid or both
  - o Lacerations easier to identify and diagnose with CT

Imaging Recommendations
- Lung lacerations and associated injuries are best depicted on a chest CT scan with IV contrast material
- Review lung, soft tissue and bone windows

Differential Diagnosis
Pulmonary Contusion
- Pulmonary hematoma (laceration filled with blood) and pulmonary contusion both present initially as air-space opacities
- Contusion will begin to clear into 2-4 days; laceration will not

Pathology
General
- Etiology-Pathogenesis
  - o Lung lacerations produced by both blunt and penetrating trauma
    - Blunt trauma causes shearing forces and tissue stresses that tear the lung parenchyma
    - Penetrating trauma directly lacerates the lung parenchyma
  - o If the laceration communicates with the pleural surface, a bronchopulmonary fistula may result

Grading
- Four types of lung lacerations have been described

Lung Laceration

- o Compression rupture: Laceration within the lung parenchyma from chest wall compression producing a rupture of the air-containing lung
- o Compression shear: Laceration in a paravertebral location due to a shear injury from sudden shifting of lower lobe across the spine
- o Rib penetration tear: Small peripheral laceration close to the chest wall where a fractured rib has punctured the lung
- o Adhesion tear: Laceration at the lung periphery due to a pre-existing adhesion limiting shifting of the lung with trauma

Clinical Issues
Presentation
- Hemoptysis, chest pain, dyspnea

Natural History
- Most lung lacerations heal well without specific treatment

Treatment
- Conservative management
- Antibiotics if laceration becomes infected

Prognosis
- Most pulmonary lacerations are of little clinical significance and heal on conservative management
- As compared with contusions which resolve within a week, lacerations take weeks to months to heal, and may result in residual pulmonary scars
- A laceration may become secondarily infected

Selected References
1. Haxhija EQ et al: Lung contusion-lacerations after blunt thoracic trauma in children. Pediatr Surg Int. 2004
2. Wagner RB et al: Classification of parenchymal injuries of the lung. Radiology 167:77-83, 1988
3. Wiot JF: The radiologic manifestations of blunt chest trauma. JAMA 231:500-3, 1975

Tracheal Laceration

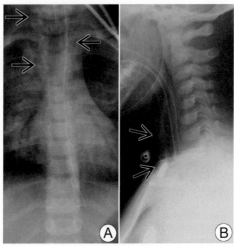

Tracheal laceration. (A) Chest film shows subcutaneous and mediastinal emphysema (arrows) as well as bilateral central pulmonary opacities. (B) Lateral view of neck shows subcutaneous emphysema (arrows) anterior to the trachea.

Key Facts
- Synonym(s): Tracheobronchial injury, tracheobronchial tear
- Definition: Laceration or transection of trachea or a main bronchus
- Classic imaging appearance
  - Pneumomediastinum on chest films
  - Subcutaneous emphysema on neck films
  - "Fallen lung" on chest films
  - Pneumothorax which does not resolve with adequate chest tube placement and suction
  - CT demonstration of a tracheal or bronchial laceration or transection
- Other key facts
  - Associated with significant chest trauma
  - Diagnosis usually confirmed with bronchoscopy

Imaging Findings
General Features
- Best imaging clue: Pneumomediastinum in a trauma patient
- Anatomy: Tracheal lacerations usually vertical at junction of cartilagenous and membranous portions of trachea
  - Bronchial lacerations/transections usually occur within 2.5 cm of carina
  - Equal incidence of injury of the right and left mainstem bronchi
Chest Film Findings
- Mediastinal emphysema with tracheal injury
- Mediastinal emphysema and/or pneumothorax with bronchial injury
- Subcutaneous emphysema
- Persistent pneumothorax despite adequate chest tube placement and suction with mainstem bronchus injury
- "Fallen lung" sign with mainstem bronchus transection
  - Lung droops to a dependent portion of chest in either supine or upright patient rather than collapsing centrally

Tracheal Laceration

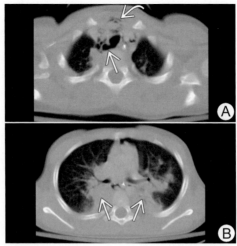

Tracheal laceration. (A) Axial CT scan of upper chest shows a tracheal laceration (arrow) at right membranous-cartilagenous junction of trachea. Curved arrow indicates pneumomediastinum anterior to trachea. (B) Axial CT scan just below carina shows bilateral air-space opacification (arrows) due to aspirated blood.

- With tracheal laceration inflated endotracheal balloon may over distend beyond expected diameter of trachea
- Tip of endotracheal tube may be extraluminal

Neck Film Findings
- Subcutaneous emphysema
- With trachea transection may see elevation of hyoid bones
  - Hyoid bones elevated above C3 level

CT Findings
- Mediastinal emphysema with tracheal injury
- Mediastinal emphysema and/or pneumothorax with bronchial injury
- Subcutaneous emphysema
- Persistent pneumothorax despite adequate chest tube placement and suction
- "Fallen lung" sign
- Identification of tracheal laceration or transection as tracheal irregularity or disruption
- Identification of bronchial laceration or transection as bronchial irregularity or disruption

Imaging Recommendations
- Chest film
  - If chest film shows pneumomediastinum perform CT
- CT scan of neck and chest with IV contrast material
- Review axial scans with soft tissue and lung windows
  - Coronal, sagittal, 3D reformations of airways may also be helpful

Differential Diagnosis
Pneumomediastium/Subcutaneous Emphysema from Other Cause
- Mediastinal and subcutaneous emphysema may also arise from pneumothorax, lung laceration, esophageal injury

Tracheal Laceration

- CT scan or bronchoscopy will exclude tracheobronchial injury
- CT scan can confirm occult pneumothorax or lung laceration
- Contrast esophagram can confirm or exclude esophageal injury

Pneumothorax From Other Cause
- Pneumothorax without bronchial laceration should resolve on chest tube suction

Pathology
General
- General Path Comments
  - Trachea lacerations often vertical at junction of membranous and cartilagenous portions of the trachea
    - A tracheal laceration may extend for several centimeters
  - Mainstem bronchi lacerations or transections usually occur adjacent to the carina
- Etiology-Pathogenesis
  - Blunt or penetrating chest trauma
  - May result from traumatic endotracheal tube placement
- Epidemiology
  - 0.4-1.5% incidence in clinical series of trauma victims
  - 2.8-5.4% incidence in autopsy series of trauma victims
  - Usually occurs in presence of other injuries

Clinical Issues
Presentation
- Tracheobronchial injuries cause impaired ventilation without overt airway obstruction
- Strider
- Hemoptysis
- Decreased oxygenation
- Persistent pneumothorax after chest tube placement (air leak) with mainstem bronchus injury
- High association with fractures of first three ribs, clavicle, sternum and scapula
- Diagnosis confirmed with bronchoscopy

Natural History
- Unrecognized tracheal injuries may lead to tracheal stenosis
- Unrecognized, bronchial injuries may lead to bronchial stenosis, bronchiectasis, atelectasis and pulmonary fibrosis

Treatment & Prognosis
- Initial selective intubation and ventilation beyond the site of injury
- Thoracotomy with surgical repair
- Good with rapid diagnosis and treatment

Selected References
1. Mason JP et al: Imaging of acute tracheobronchial injury: review of the literature. Emerg Med 1:250-60, 1994
2. Unger JM et al: Tears of the trachea and main bronchi caused by blunt trauma: radiologic findings. AJR 153:1175-80, 1989
3. Halttunen PE et al: Bronchial rupture caused by blunt chest trauma. Scan J Cardiovasc Surg. 18:141-4, 1984

Aortic Trauma

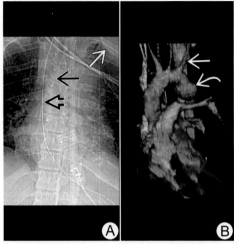

Aortic trauma. (A) Chest film shows displacement of nasogastric tube (open arrow) and trachea (black arrow) to right. Aortic shadow is enlarged. Left apical cap (white arrow). (B) 3D CT of aorta shows traumatic false aneurysm (curved arrow) just beyond left subclavian artery (arrow).

Key Facts
- Synonym(s): Aortic injury, traumatic false aneurysm of aorta, traumatic aortic disruption
- Definition: Injury of the thoracic aorta
- Classic imaging appearance
  - Mediastinal widening on chest film
  - Mediastinal hemorrhage and aortic injury at CT
- Other key facts
  - Aortic injury at junction of posterior aortic arch and proximal descending aorta
  - Life-threatening injury responsible for 15-20% of motor vehicle fatalities
  - Normal chest film nearly excludes aortic trauma
  - Quickly and accurately diagnosed by CT
  - CT shows both aortic injury and mediastinal hemorrhage

Imaging Findings
<u>General Features</u>
- Best imaging clue
  - Mediastinal widening on chest film
<u>Chest Film Findings</u>
- Mediastinal widening
- Displacement of nasogastric tube to the right
- Displacement of endotracheal tube to the right
- Enlargement of aortic arch shadow
- Loss of definition of aortic arch
- Left apical cap representing extrapleural hemorrhage
<u>CT Findings</u>
- Indirect sign (mediastinal finding)
  - Mediastinal hemorrhage

Aortic Trauma

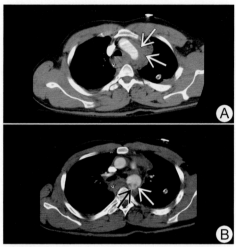

Aortic trauma. (A) Axial CT scan through level of aortic arch shows mediastinal hemorrhage (arrows) around the arch. (B) Axial CT scan through the level of aortic injury shows intimal disruption (arrows) with intraluminal flaps and thrombus.

- With aortic injury usually adjacent to aorta at junction of posterior arch and proximal descending aorta
- Isolated anterior mediastinal hematoma usually not caused by aortic injury
- Direct signs (aortic findings)
  - Aortic contour abnormality
  - Intimal flap or disruption
  - False aneurysm formation
  - Abrupt tapering of the aorta (pseudocoarctation)
  - Thrombus or debris protruding into aortic lumen
  - Extravasation of IV contrast material

Aortography Findings
- The "gold standard" for aortic trauma diagnosis
  - Less commonly used today
- Will show all aortic findings mentioned above
- Aortography preferred for suspected injury of brachiocephalic arteries

Imaging Recommendations
- Chest film
  - Normal chest film virtually excludes aortic trauma
  - If chest film abnormal, perform CT
- Chest CT with IV contrast material
  - Review mediastinum and aorta on axial slices
  - Perform CTA if injury present
    - Show relationship between injury and left subclavian artery
  - Search for other chest injuries
- Aortography
  - Usually definitive if CT scan is indeterminate

Aortic Trauma

Differential Diagnosis
Mediastinal Widening From Other Causes
- Hemorrhage from sternal fracture, sternoclavicular dislocation, thoracic spine fracture, injury to mediastinal venous structure
- Mediastinal widening from tortuous blood vessels, residual thymus, lymphadenopathy, mediastinal lipomatosis
- CT will show no evidence of aortic injury

Pathology
General
- General Path Comments
  - Usually involves proximal descending aorta just beyond origin of left subclavian artery
  - In surviving patients, injury consists of an intimal tear of aortic wall with hemorrhage contained by adventia and surrounding soft tissues
    - Forms a periaortic hematoma
- Etiology
  - Rapid deceleration resulting in differential forces on the proximal descending aorta between fixed and more mobile segments
- Epidemiology
  - 8,000 cases per year in USA
  - Accounts for 15-20% of all motor vehicle collision fatalities
  - 90% die before reaching the hospital

Clinical Issues
Presentation
- Multiple trauma patient in deceleration accident
- Multiple organ injury often present
Natural History
- High morbidity and mortality if untreated due to massive hemorrhage
Treatment
- Initial temporizing measures including fluid therapy, hemodynamic monitoring and blood pressure control
- Aortic surgery or intervention
  - Thoracotomy with aortic graft or primary repair
  - Percutaneous placement of an aortic endovascular stent
Prognosis
- Good with rapid diagnosis and treatment
- Prognosis also related to the extent of other injuries

Selected Reference
1.   Gavant Ml et al: Blunt traumatic aortic rupture: Detection with helical CT of the chest. Radiology 197:125-33, 1995
2.   Williams JS et al: Aortic injury in vehicular trauma. Ann Thorac Surg 57:726-30, 1994
3.   Mirvis SE et al: Value of chest radiography in excluding aortic rupture. Radiology 163:487-93, 1987

Diaphragm Rupture

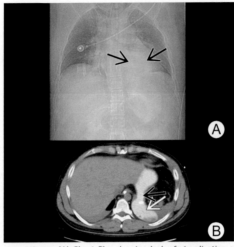

Left diaphragm rupture. (A) Chest film showing lack of visualization of the medial aspect of the left hemidiaphragm. Black arrows indicate increased retrocardiac density representing a herniated stomach. (B) Axial CT scan showing herniation of the stomach (white arrow) into the chest. Black arrow indicates the collar sign.

Key Facts
- Synonym(s): Diaphragm tear, traumatic herniation of the stomach
- Definition
  - Traumatic laceration or tear of the diaphragm usually associated with herniation of abdominal viscera into the chest
- Classic imaging appearance
  - Abdominal viscera located above the diaphragm
- Other key facts
  - Caused by penetrating or blunt trauma
  - Left-sided injuries more common
  - Diagnosis of herniated abdominal viscera may be immediate or delayed months to years after the injury

Imaging Findings
General Features
- Best imaging clue
  - Visualization of abdominal viscera above the diaphragm

Chest Film Findings
- Majority of patients have an abnormal chest film
- Hemothorax
- Pneumothorax
- Loss of visualization of the diaphragm
- Basel pulmonary opacity
- Apparent elevation of the diaphragm
- Upward extension of the nasogastric tube above the diaphragm
- Stomach or bowel above the diaphragm
- Shift of the mediastinum to the opposite side

Bowel Contrast Examination
- Upper GI series or barium enema may show stomach or bowel above the diaphragm

Diaphragm Rupture

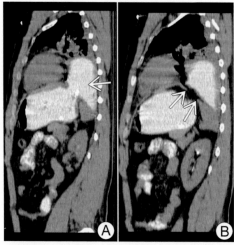

Left diaphragm rupture. (A) Sagittal CT reformation through left hemidiaphragm. Arrow indicates herniated stomach in the left chest. (B) Slightly more medial sagittal reformation. Arrows indicate a discontinuity of the diaphragm at the site of rupture.

CT Findings
- Collar sign of herniated stomach, bowel or liver extending above the diaphragm
  - Collar sign refers to a waist-like constriction of herniated viscera at the site of herniation
- Stomach, loops of bowel or mesentery above the diaphragm
- Coronal and sagittal reformations can show discontinuity the diaphragm and herniated abdominal viscera

MR Findings
- Focal discontinuities of the diaphragm well shown on coronal and sagittal MR images
- On T1 sequences the hyperintense abdominal and mediastinal fat permit optimal visualization of the hypointense diaphragm

Imaging Recommendations
- Chest-abdomen CT scans with oral and IV contrast materials and with coronal and sagittal CT reformations
- Coronal and sagittal T1-weighted MR scans

Differential Diagnosis
- Loss of visualization of the diaphragm due to hemothorax, or to atelectasis or air-space disease at the lung base

Pathology
General
- General Path Comments
  - Reported increase frequency of left side rupture although right-sided injuries often remain under diagnosed
  - With right-sided injury the liver may protect against significant organ herniation into the right thorax

- o Most ruptures involve the posteriorlateral portion of diaphragm near the junction of the central tendon and posterior leaves
- o Visceral herniation occurs in 95% of left sided injuries but may be delayed and not recognized until later
- o The stomach is the most frequent organ to herniate
- Etiology-Pathogenesis
  - o Penetrating trauma is the most common cause of diaphragmatic injury
  - o Rupture with blunt trauma is caused by a sudden increase in intrathoracic or intra-abdominal pressure against a fixed diaphragm
    - ▪ Injuries from blunt trauma are more often associated with large ruptures and herniated viscera
    - ▪ Injuries from penetrating trauma are usually small
- Epidemiology
  - o Diaphragmatic injuries seen in about 5% of patients undergoing laparotomy or thoracotomy for trauma

Clinical Issues
Presentation
- Chest pain
- Decreased ventilation
- Bowel sounds in the chest
- Mediastinal shift

Natural History
- If not diagnosed and treated the patient may remain asymptomatic or may later develop incarceration of herniated abdominal viscera

Treatment
- Laparotomy with reduction of herniated structures and transabdominal diaphragm repair
- Right thoracotomy may be required to facilitate repair of a right-sided rupture

Prognosis
- Patients undergoing early diagnosis and repair do very well
- If the diagnosis is initially overlooked, patient may later experience incarceration of herniated viscera

Selected References
1. Iochum S et al: Imaging of diaphragmatic injury: A diagnostic challenge. Radiographics. 22:103-18, 2002
2. Killeen KL et al: Helical CT of diaphragmatic rupture caused by blunt trauma. AJR. 173:1611-6, 1999
3. Shah R et al: Traumatic rupture of the diaphragm. Ann Thorac Surg. 60:1444-9, 1995

Cardiac Injury

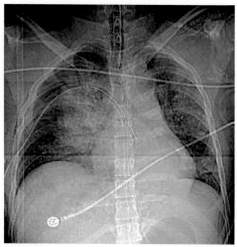

Cardiac rupture with hemopericardium. AP chest film of blunt trauma patient who suffered steering wheel injury to chest. Peri-hilar haziness & patchy lung opacities are seen representing pulmonary contusion & pulmonary edema. Heart is slightly globular in shape. Right chest tube placed for a right pneumothorax.

Key Facts
- Synonym(s): Cardiac trauma, cardiac rupture
- Definition: Injury to heart caused by blunt or penetrating trauma
- Classic imaging appearance
  - Globular appearance of heart due to presence of hemopericardium; hemopericardium on CT
- Other key facts
  - Consider cardiac injury in trauma patients with abnormal EKG tracings &/or clinical signs of pericardial tamponade
  - Cardiac injury, especially rupture, is highly lethal & prompt diagnosis & treatment is required for a favorable outcome
  - Associated with anterior blows to chest
  - Associated with sternal fractures

Imaging Findings
General Features
- Best imaging clues: Globular heart on chest film; thickening of pericardial space at CT
  - Fluid in pericardial space will measure blood density (> 40 HU)
  - Sternal fracture
- Anatomy: Cardiac injuries more commonly involve right atrium & right ventricle
Chest Film Findings
- Globular heart; pulmonary edema; hemothorax; sternal fracture or other signs of chest trauma
CT Findings
- Hemopericardium; pneumopericardium; anterior mediastinal hematoma directly in front of heart

Cardiac Injury

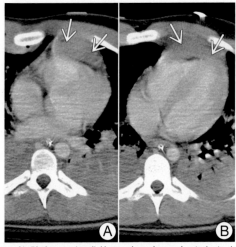

Chest CT scans (A, B) show pericardial hemorrhage (arrows) anterior to right ventricle. Bilateral hemothoraces & subcutaneous emphysema are present. Patient developed clinical signs of pericardial tamponade. At thoracotomy a laceration was found & repaired at junction of right atrium & right ventricle.

TEE (Transthoracic Echocardiogram)
- Can detect pericardial effusion, myocardial contusion, valvular disruption or abnormal cardiac function

Imaging Recommendations
- Chest film; chest CT scan with IV contrast material; TEE

Differential Diagnosis

Pericardial Effussion
- Fluid in pericardial space measures water density (< 10 HU)

Myocardiac Infarction
- Trauma patient with abnormal EKG tracing due cardiac ischemia rather than cardiac trauma: No hemopericardium

Myocardial Contusion
- Abnormal EKG & TEE but no major hemorrhage

Pathology

General
- General Path Comments
  - Heart is well protected from most blunt trauma
  - Most cardiac injuries result from penetrating trauma
  - Severe blunt chest trauma may produce cardiac contusion, cardiac rupture, pneumopericardium, hemopericardium, cardiac tamponade & cardiac valve rupture
  - Cardiac ruptures usually involve right atrium or right ventricle & may bleed into pericardium or anterior mediastinum
  - Rapid accumulation of blood (hemopericardium) or air (pneumopericardium) in pericardial sac may lead cardiac tamponade
- Etiology-Pathogenesis

Cardiac Injury

- o Penetrating cardiac injuries from stab wounds & gun shots
- o Cardiac injuries from blunt trauma associated with anterior chest wall trauma
  - ▪ From impact of steering wheel in motor vehicle collisions
  - ▪ High association with sternal fractures
- Epidemiology
  - o 10% incidence of cardiac injury in autopsy series of chest trauma patients
  - o Cardiac rupture from blunt trauma accounts for 5% of 50,000 annual highway deaths in US

Gross Pathologic-Surgical Features
- Blunt trauma may injure myocardium, valves or coronary arteries
- All four chambers are susceptible to rupture although ventricular ruptures predominate
  - o Ventricular rupture usually from direct anterior blow to chest
  - o Blows that produce sudden increase in preload can cause atrial rupture
  - o Penetrating trauma may involve any chamber

Clinical Issues
Presentation
- Depends on site of rupture & integrity of pericardium
  - o 30% have concomitant pericardial laceration with exsanguination into mediastinum or hemithorax, 70% have initial pericardial tamponade
- With pericardial tamponade patients present Beck's triad
  - o Jugular vein distension
    - ▪ Due to elevated central venous pressure
  - o Muffled heart sounds, hypotension or shock
- With myocardial laceration patients remain hypotensive in spite of fluid therapy
- Cardiac injuries suspected when EKG changes occur in setting of blunt trauma

Natural History
- Cardiac rupture with hemopericardium may be fatal due to pericardial tamponade or exsanguination into thorax
- Majority of deaths occur before patients arrive at a hospital
- Untreated valvular injury may lead to cardiac failure

Treatment & Prognosis
- Initial management with rapid evacuation of pericardial blood via pericardiocentesis or subxiphoid pericardial window
- Myocardial laceration requires emergency thoracostomy for relief of tamponade & repair of myocardial injury
- Myocardial contusion usually responds to conservative measures and is rarely associated with significant cardiac failure of arrhythmias
- Variable related to type of cardiac injury
- Cardiac rupture has a high mortality rate
  - o Survival is more common with right-sided injuries, especially right atrial rupture

Selected References
1. Stern EJ et al: Acute traumatic Hemopericardium. AJR. 162:1305-6, 1994
2. Mirvis SE et al: Posttraumatic tension pneumopericardium: The "small heart" sign. Radiology. 158:663-9, 1986

PocketRadiologist®
ER-Trauma
Top 100 Diagnoses

ABDOMINAL INJURY

Hemoperitoneum

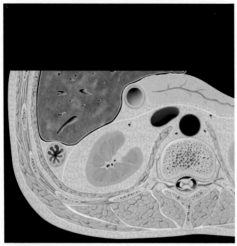

Intraperitoneal blood may surround the inferior tip of the liver. In contrast, the anterior renal fascia merges with the lateral conal fascia thus preventing blood in the anterior pararenal space from accumulating lateral to the liver. This helps differentiate hemoperitoneum from blood in the retroperitoneal space.

Key Facts
- Definition: Free blood within the peritoneal cavity
- Classic imaging appearance: Fluid within the various peritoneal spaces which is not contained within a viscus
- Other key facts
  - The peritoneal cavities and spaces in which free blood may be seen include the perisplenic and perihepatic spaces, Morrison's pouch, pericolic gutters, inframesocolic space, interloop collections within the mesentery, and pelvis
  - The density of blood is usually greater than 30 HU
    - Clotted blood is 40-75 HU
    - Unclotted blood is 25-50 HU
    - Blood may mix with other fluid present and be of lower density
  - Volume of blood may be characterized as mild, moderate, or major
    - Mild: One compartment; 100-200 mL
    - Moderate: Two compartments; 250-500 mL
    - Major: Greater than two compartments; > 500 mL
  - Free blood signifies injury to
    - Solid organs
    - Hollow viscus
    - Vessels

Imaging Findings
General Features
- Best imaging clue: With plain films, air containing bowel floats toward the center of the abdomen, there is increased haziness of the film, soft tissue density may be seen between the colon and properitoneal fat (widening of the flank stripe)
CT Findings
- The density of free blood will be as indicated above

149

Hemoperitoneum

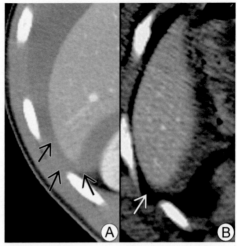

(A) Free intraperitoneal blood wraps around the tip of the liver (arrows). (B) Blood in the anterior pararenal space due to a laceration of the bare area of the liver is seen posterior to the liver, is confined to the anterior pararenal space and does not accumulate lateral to the liver (arrow).

- Intraperitoneal blood will wrap around the tip of the liver
  - Retroperitoneal blood, in contrast, is confined by the fusion of the anterior pararenal fascia with the lateral conal fascia and may appear subhepatic but does not wrap around the tip of the liver

Imaging Recommendations
- CT should be performed instead of, or prior to peritoneal lavage if possible
- Imaging in trauma should always include both the abdomen and pelvis, since free blood may accumulate only in the pelvis, yet be a clue to upper abdominal injury
- Hemoperitoneum is evaluated during routine CT for trauma which includes 5 mm thick images and 5 mm image spacing, using an injection rate of at least 2.5 mL/sec for 135-180 mL of contrast, and using a 75 sec delay after beginning injection until starting the scan at the dome of the diaphragm

Differential Diagnosis
Other Free Fluid
- Urine, chyle, bile, lavage fluid and bowel content may accumulate in the intraperitoneal spaces and be seen as free fluid.
  - Pure non-bloody free fluid will be 5-10 HU
  - Peritoneal lavage may be useful after CT to differentiate the type of fluid which is present

Pathology
- None relevant to this case

Hemoperitoneum

Clinical Issues

<u>Presentation</u>
- After large extravascular bleeding into the peritoneal cavity, patients may appear hypotensive
- Hemoperitoneum may lead to symptoms of peritonitis and cause a febrile response in the post trauma period and mimic infection
- Isolated free fluid in stable patients without an apparent source from an injury can be seen in 2-3% of patients
  - Management of the patient with this isolated finding is variable and includes diagnostic lavage, observation, laparotomy or repeat CT

<u>Natural History</u>
- Free intraperitoneal blood usually resorbs without sequellae

Selected References
1. Rodriguez et al: Isolated free fluid on computed tomographic scan in blunt abdominal trauma: a systematic review of incidence and management. J Trauma;53:79-85, 2002
2. Ochsner MG: Factors of failure for nonoperative management of blunt liver and splenic injuries. World J Surg. 25:1393-6, 2001
3. Novelline RA et al: Helical CT in emergency radiology. Radiology. 213:321-39, 1999

Active Intraperitoneal Bleed

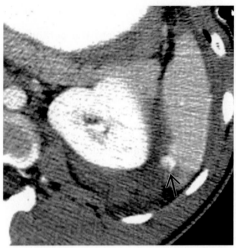

Active bleeding from the spleen is noted (arrow). There is also a small amount of blood seen anterior to the spleen. The blood posterior to the kidney is unrelated to the splenic injury, which results in intraperitoneal bleeding or bleeding within the spleen itself.

Key Facts
- Definition: Active bleeding is seen as extravasation of high density IV contrast material outside the confines of a blood vessel
- Classic imaging appearance: Contrast tends to pool at the site of injury and is seen as a high density collection
  - Bleeding may be seen as a rounded, linear, curvilinear or amorphous collection adjacent to or within the injured organ
- Other key facts
  - Active bleeding is seen in 13-18% of CT scans for blunt abdominal trauma
  - Active bleeding is most frequently seen in spleen or liver, since these are most frequently injured organs; most frequent organs to show active bleeding if they are injured are the kidney and mesentery
  - Intervention with surgery or embolization is about three times as frequent if active bleeding is seen

Imaging Findings
General Features
- Best imaging clue: Extravascular contrast material noted during arterial phase or on delayed images
CT Findings
- On non-contrast CT active bleeding is the same density as blood in the organs or vessels, and is not readily identified; clot may form near the site of injury which appears of higher density than surrounding organs or free blood (the sentinal clot sign)
- Contrast enhanced CT will show extraluminal contrast

Active Intraperitoneal Bleed

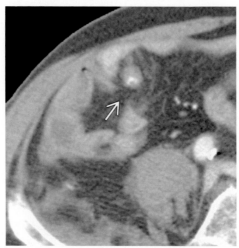

Active bleeding was found at surgery from a mesenteric artery in right lower quadrant. Arrow indicates an amorphous collection of contrast within mesentery. The collection is larger than adjacent vessels.

<u>Imaging Recommendations</u>
- Active bleeding is best detected on contrast enhanced CT using 5 mm thick images and 5 mm image spacing, using an injection rate of at least 2.5 mL/sec for 135-180 mL of contrast, & using a 75 sec delay after beginning injection until starting the scan at dome of diaphragm

Differential Diagnosis
- None relevant to this case

Pathology
- None relevant to this case

Clinical Issues
<u>Presentation</u>
- Patients with active arterial extravasation more likely to be hypotensive
<u>Treatment</u>
- Surgery, embolization or close observation is needed if active bleeding is noted
  - o The decision to intervene is based on the stability of the patient
<u>Prognosis</u>
- Outcome is favorable if the active arterial bleeding can be controlled
- Control of bleeding is more difficult in areas of problematic access such as the retrohepatic region

Selected References
1. Willmann et al: Multidetector CT: Detection of active hemorrhage in patients with blunt abdominal trauma. AJR Am J Roentgenol 179:437-44, 2002
2. Yao et al: Using contrast-enhanced helical CT to visualize arterial extravasation after blunt abdominal trauma: Incidence and organ distribution. AJR Am J Roentgenol 178:17-20, 2002
3. Shanmuganathan K et al: Nonsurgical management of blunt splenic injury: Use of CT criteria to select patients for splenic arteriography and potential endovascular therapy. Radiology 217:75-82, 2000

Splenic Trauma

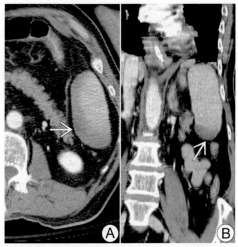

(A) Blood is surrounding medial surface of spleen (arrow). Subcapsular hematomas usually cause an indentation of splenic parenchyma; either flattening or a concave impression. (B) Coronal CT reformation shows subcapsular hematoma to be located at inferior pole of spleen there is flattening not seen on axial images (arrow).

Key Facts
- Definition: Damage to the splenic parenchyma or splenic vessels secondary to blunt or penetrating trauma
- Other key facts
  - Spleen is most commonly injured organ following blunt trauma
    - Spleen injury accounts for about 40% of patients with blunt organ injury
  - Nonoperative management possible in about 60% of patients
    - Failure of nonoperative management increases with grade of injury
  - The only finding at CT may be perisplenic blood

Imaging Findings
General Features
- Types of injury
  - Laceration
    - Linear or curved area of low attenuation relative to spleen
  - Intrasplenic hematoma
    - Rounded inhomogeneous area of low attenuation
  - Subcapsular hematoma
    - Crescentic low attenuation area compressing the parenchyma
  - Fracture
    - Multiple crossing lacerations or fragmentation
  - Hilar vascular injury
    - Devascularized splenic segment or devascularized whole spleen

CT Findings
- In addition to the above findings, CT may show the following, of which both increase the likelihood of intervention
  - Active bleeding

Splenic Trauma

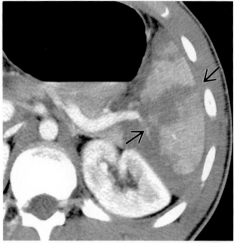

There is a fracture of the spleen; a through and through laceration is present (arrows). There is fragmentation and the fracture extends to the splenic hilum. This would be a grade V injury.

o Expanding hematoma on a follow-up scan

Imaging Recommendations
- Splenic injury is evaluated during routine CT for trauma which includes detector configuration of (e.g.,) 4 x 2.5 mm, 15 mm/sec table speed, 5 mm thick images and 5 mm image spacing, using an injection rate of at least 2.5 mL/sec for 135-180 mL of contrast, and using a 75 sec delay after beginning injection until starting the scan at the dome of the diaphragm
- Delayed scanning may be useful if there is active arterial hemorrhage
- Follow-up scan may be useful if patient is suspected of having continued bleeding from expanding hematoma or rupture of the spleen

Differential Diagnosis
- None

Pathology
Staging or Grading Criteria
- Subcapsular hematoma
  o Grade I: < 10% surface area
  o Grade II: 10-50%
  o Grade III: > 50% or expanding
- Intraparenchymal hematoma
  o Grade II: < 5 cm diameter
  o Grade III: > 5 cm or expanding
- Laceration
  o Grade I: < 1 cm in length
  o Grade II: 1-3 cm
  o Grade III: > 3cm
- Devascularization

- o Grade IV: > 25% of splenic area
- o Grade V: Total spleen
- Shattered spleen (fragmentation, multiple fractures)
  - o Grade V

Clinical Issues

Presentation
- Acute injury may lead to hypotension and a drop in hematocrit; delayed rupture will also present in this way

Treatment
- Surgery is required if the patient becomes hemodynamically unstable after initial stabilization
- Predictors of failure of nonoperative management
  - o Onset of homodynamic instability
  - o Injury grade IV or V
  - o Large associated hemoperitoneum
  - o Active arterial extravasation seen on CT

Prognosis
- Complications following nonoperative management
  - o "Delayed rupture" weeks to years after initial injury; seen in < 1% of patients if initial CT is normal
  - o Pseudoaneurysm
  - o Pseudocyst; if > 5 cm there is 25% risk of rupture
  - o Abscess which may be delayed months or years

Selected References
1. Nance ML et al: Pattern of abdominal free fluid following isolated blunt splenic or liver injury in the pediatric patient. J Trauma 52:85-7, 2002
2. Yao DC et al: Using contrast enhanced helical CT to visualize arterial extravasation after blunt abdominal trauma: Incidence and organ distribution. AJR 178:17-20, 2002
3. Uecker J et al: The role of follow up radiographic studies in non-operative management of splenic trauma. Am Surg. 67:22-5, 2001

Hepatic Injury

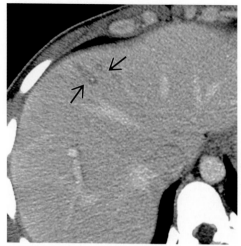

Two small hepatic lacerations are seen (arrows). These appear of lower CT attenuation than the surrounding liver, which is perfused with contrast. This would constitute a grade II injury since the laceration is about 2 cm long.

Key Facts
- Definition: Hepatic injury is seen as damage to the hepatic parenchyma or blood vessels
- Other key facts
  - Liver injury occurs in 15-20% of patients with blunt trauma
  - Associated injuries occur in 65% of patients with penetrating trauma and 50% of those with blunt trauma (frequently splenic injury)
  - Nonoperative management is successful in about 80% of adults and over 90% of children

Imaging Findings
General Features
- Types of injury
  - Hematoma: Subcapsular, intraparenchymal
    - Rounded inhomogeneous area of low attenuation within parenchyma, or crescentic low attenuation area compressing the parenchyma
  - Contusion
    - Area of low attenuation relative to parenchyma
  - Laceration: Linear, stellate
    - Linear or curved area of low attenuation relative to liver
  - Fracture
    - Multiple crossing lacerations or fragmentation
  - Venous, arterial or biliary injury
    - Extravasation of bile or blood, poor perfusion of involved liver segment
- Anatomy
  - Posteriorly located "bare area" of liver is not covered by peritoneum but communicates directly with the retroperitoneum

Hepatic Injury

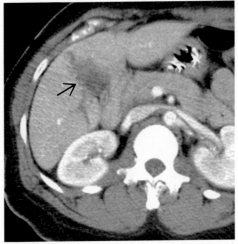

Intraparenchymal hematoma (arrow) extending near the porta within the liver would be a grade II or III injury.

- Laceration in bare area can produce blood in the anterior pararenal space instead of intraperitoneal blood

CT Findings
- In addition to the above findings CT may show
  - Active bleeding
  - Expanding hematoma on a follow-up CT scan

Imaging Recommendations
- Hepatic injury is evaluated during routine CT for trauma which includes detector configuration of (e.g.,) 4 x 2.5 mm, 15 mm/sec table speed, 5mm thick images and 5 mm image spacing, using an injection rate of at least 2.5 mL/sec for 135-180 mL of contrast, and using a 75 sec delay after beginning injection until starting the scan at the dome of the diaphragm
- Delayed scanning may be useful if there is a parenchymal organ injury to search for active arterial hemorrhage
- With instability of the patient, embolization is an option

Differential Diagnosis
- None relevant to this case

Pathology

Staging or Grading Criteria
- Hematoma (subcapsular or parenchymal)
  - Grade I: < 1 cm diameter
  - Grade II: 1-3 cm
  - Grade III: > 3 cm
- Laceration
  - Grade I: < 1 cm deep
  - Grade II: 1-3 cm
  - Grade III: > 3 cm

- Parenchymal disruption
  - Grade IV: 25-75% of hepatic lobe, 1-3 segments
  - Grade V: > 75% of hepatic lobe, > 3 segments
- Juxtahepatic venous injury
  - Grade V: Interior vena cava or central hepatic vein injury

Clinical Issues
Presentation
- Multitrauma patient with abdominal symptoms or signs, possible hypotension and low hematocrit
Treatment
- Difficult injury to treat surgically because of uncontrolled bleeding, especially in children, led to more conservative therapy
- Patients with hemostatic disorder, active arterial extravasation, or grade IV or V injuries, especially with injury to main trunks of hepatic veins, are more likely to fail supportive therapy and require embolization or surgery
  - About 13% of patients with liver injury sustain injury to hepatic veins
Prognosis
- Mortality of 10-15% overall
- Mortality of 50-80% with juxtahepatic venous injury
- Complications following nonoperative management include
  - Intrahepatic vascular fistulas
  - Delayed hemorrhage
  - Bilomas
  - Abscess
  - Hyperpyrexia from large hemoperitoneum
  - Posttraumatic liver cyst

Selected References
1. Carrillo EH et al: Evolution in the treatment of complex blunt liver injuries. Curr Probl Surg. 38:1-60, 2001
2. Poletti PA et al: CT criteria for management of blunt liver trauma: Correlation with angiographic and surgical findings. Radiology. 216:418-27, 2000
3. Shanmuganathan K et al: CT scan evaluation of blunt hepatic trauma. Radiol Clin North Am. 36:399-411, 1998

Gallbladder/Biliary Injury

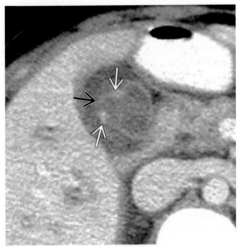

Gallbladder rupture was found at surgery with active bleeding from the wall of the gallbladder. At CT a segment the wall of the gallbladder is not seen (black arrow) and high-density contrast is noted extravasating from the injured wall (white arrows). There is pericholecystic fluid consistent with blood.

Key Facts
- Definition: Abnormalities of the gallbladder wall, content or pericholecystic region following trauma
- Other key facts
  - Gallbladder injury occurs in only 2-8% of patients with blunt trauma since the gallbladder is relatively protected by the liver
  - Extrahepatic bile duct injury occurs about ¼ as frequently as gallbladder injury
  - Associated injuries are frequent
    - Liver in 80%
    - Duodenum in 50%

Imaging Findings
General Features
- Other generic features: Three types of injury may be seen
  - Wall contusion
  - Rupture
  - Avulsion
CT Findings
- Wall abnormalities
  - Wall thickening
  - Irregular ill-defined wall contour
  - Mucosal flap
- Gallbladder content abnormality
  - Collapsed lumen
  - High density content of gallbladder (blood mixed with bile)
- Other findings
  - Pericholecystic fluid consisting of blood or blood mixed with bile; the density of this fluid will be variable
  - Active arterial extravasation of IV contrast material

Gallbladder/Biliary Injury

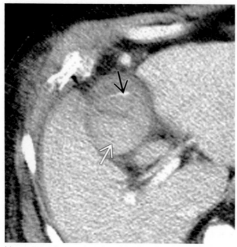

The gallbladder content is noted to be of higher density than would be expected. This high-density content would reflect unopacified blood mixed with bile (white arrow). In this patient there is active arterial extravasation (black arrow) noted into the lumen.

- o Bile duct injury will result in extravasation of bile near the injured duct

<u>Imaging Recommendations</u>
- Gallbladder injury is best detected on contrast enhanced CT using 5 mm thick images and 5 mm image spacing, using an injection rate of at least 2.5 mL/sec for 135-180 mL of contrast, and using a 75 sec delay after beginning injection until starting the scan at the dome of the diaphragm

Differential Diagnosis
<u>Periportal Tracking</u>
- Periportal tracking refers to zones of low density fluid surrounding the bile ducts and vessels within the liver parenchyma
  - o Diffuse tracking may occur in patients with fluid overload following resuscitation; bile duct injury usually results in a more focal area of tracking

<u>Pericholecystic Fluid</u>
- Pericholecystic fluid alone may occur from various factors unrelated to gallbladder injury: Fluid overload, ascites, CHF, or adjacent liver injury

Pathology
<u>General</u>
- Wall rupture may be seen in the resected specimen

Clinical Issues
<u>Presentation</u>
- There is no acute specific finding that would suggest gallbladder or biliary injury
- Bile in the peritoneal cavity may result in peritonitis

Gallbladder/Biliary Injury

<u>Treatment</u>
- Gallbladder injury may require surgery if there is rupture or avulsion of the gallbladder
- Wall contusion may be treated conservatively
- Intrahepatic bile duct injury may heal
- Extrahepatic bile duct injury may require surgery due to continued leading of bile and peritonitis

Selected References
1. Kao EY, et al: Sonographic diagnosis of traumatic gallbladder rupture. J Ultrasound Med. 21:1295-7, 2002
2. Contini S, et al: Gallbladder injury in blunt abdominal trauma. Surg Endosc. 15:757, 2001
3. Endress C, et al: Traumatic gallbladder rupture: CT diagnosis. AJR Am J Roentgenol. 165:738, 1995

Small Bowel Injury

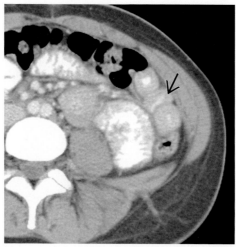

Small bowel loops are thickened (arrow). There is little other evidence of small bowel injury adjacent to this small bowel hematoma.

Key Facts
- Definition: Hematoma of the small bowel wall or perforation
- Classic imaging appearance: Bowel wall thickening with free fluid
- Other key facts
- Bowel injury occurs in about 5% of patients sustaining blunt abdominal trauma; small bowel injury occurs in about 2/3 of patients with bowel injury
- Associated injuries of adjacent viscera are frequent
  - Seat belt syndrome includes bruising of the anterior abdominal wall (seat belt sign), bowel or mesenteric injury, lumbar spine fracture, other visceral injuries
- Accuracy of diagnosis with CT
  - Recent overall accuracy: 84-99%
  - Accuracy has improved with multislice scanners
  - Bowel and pancreatic injuries more likely to be missed with CT than other injuries following blunt trauma

Imaging Findings
General Features
- Best imaging clue: Free fluid and small bowel wall thickening
- <u>CT Findings</u>
- Small bowel abnormalities
  - Bowel wall thickening of injured segment
  - Bowel wall enhancement
  - Defect in bowel wall (rarely seen)
  - Findings of bowel ischemia may occur with mesenteric artery injury
- Other findings may or may not be present
  - Free low density (10 HU) fluid
    - Interloop fluid
    - Free fluid in intraperitoneal compartments, such as pericolic gutters or pelvis

Small Bowel Injury

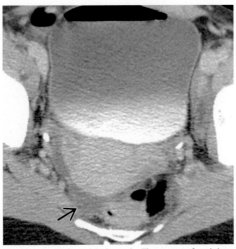

Low-density fluid is seen in the pelvis (arrow). The source of such low-density fluid could be bowel, urinary bladder, bile, preexisting ascites, or levage fluid. In this patient the only injury found was small bowel perforation. Pelvic free fluid may be the only finding of upper abdominal bowel injury.

- o Extraluminal oval contrast
- o Free air
- o Fat stranding
- o Mesenteric hematoma

Imaging Recommendations
- CT is the imaging modality of choice
- US may detect free fluid in the unstable patient but the false negative rate with US is about 40% for bowel and mesenteric injuries
- Oral contrast should be used to diagnose bowel wall thickening or contrast extravasation
- If scanning cannot be delayed for opacification of the small bowel, oral contrast is still indicated for aid in diagnosing duodenal and pancreatic injuries
- CT technique includes oral and intravenous contrast with 5 mm thick images and 5 mm image spacing, using an injection rate of at least 2.5 mL/sec for 135-180 mL of contrast, and using a 75 sec delay after beginning injection until starting the scan at the dome of the diaphragm
- CT should include both the abdomen and pelvis since the only finding of small bowel injury may be free low-density fluid within the pelvis

Differential Diagnosis
Rapid Fluid Resuscitation
- Mesenteric edema and bowel wall edema occur with fluid overload
  - o If due to rapid fluid, findings are diffuse rather than focal
  - o Other findings from rapid fluid administration, not seen with bowel injury, include
    - ▪ Diffuse retroperitoneal fluid accumulation
    - ▪ Large IVC
    - ▪ Periportal tracking

Small Bowel Injury

- Pericholecystic fluid

Shock Bowel
- Bowel wall enhancement may result from relative hypotension of bowel resulting in
  o Shunting of blood flow to the mucosa
  o Prolongation of transit time of contrast enhanced blood through bowel wall
- Other findings of shock bowel not seen with bowel injury include
  o Fluid filled and distended bowel
  o Flat IVC
  o Small aorta may be seen, especially in children

Pathology
- None relevant to this case

Clinical Issues
Presentation
- There are no specific acute signs or symptoms of bowel injury
  o Paralytic ileus, abdominal tenderness and rigidity may be identified
Treatment
- Surgery is indicated when there is bowel perforation
Prognosis
- Unrecognized injury to the vascular supply to a small bowel segment may lead to stenosis of the small bowel and delayed onset of obstruction
- Post trauma intussusception has been reported
- Obstruction due to incarceration in trauma induced hernia may occur

Selected References
1.   Killeen KL et al: Helical computed tomography of bowel and mesenteric injuries. J Trauma. 51:26-36, 2001
2.   Tsushima Y et al: Ischaemic ileal stenosis following blunt abdominal trauma and demonstrated by CT. Br J Radiol. 74:277-9, 2001
3.   Richards JR et. al: Bowel and mesenteric injury: Evaluation with emergency abdominal US. Radiology. 211:399-403, 1999

Colon Injury

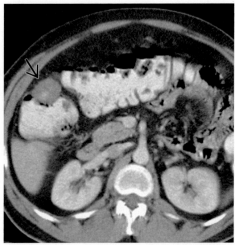

A rounded soft tissue density (arrow) is noted in antero-lateral aspect of the wall of the ascending colon. There was no bowel contrast extravasation or free air. The patient had been stabbed in the right flank. Surgery showed a bowel wall hematoma which had sealed off a through and through colonic perforation.

Key Facts
- Definition: Blunt or penetrating trauma may injure the bowel wall resulting in contusion, hematoma or perforation; interruption of arterial supply may lead to ischemia of involved segment
- Other key facts
- The bowel is injured in about 5% of patients having laparotomy after blunt trauma
  - Colon injury constitutes about 20% of bowel injuries in blunt trauma
- In penetrating trauma goal of CT is to detect evidence of peritoneal penetration, bowel, vessel, and other organ injury
  - Use of triple contrast technique in penetrating trauma is very accurate in predicting need for laparotomy
    - E.g., 100% sensitivity, 96% specificity, 100% NPV, 97% accuracy
- Associated injuries to other organs are frequent

Imaging Findings
General Features
- Best imaging clue: Colon wall abnormality and extraluminal fluid, air or bowel contrast material
CT Findings
- Colon wall abnormalities
  - Thickening
  - Enhancement of wall of injured segment
  - Discontinuity
- Other abnormalities
  - Free fluid
  - Free air, either retroperitoneal or intraperitoneal

Colon Injury

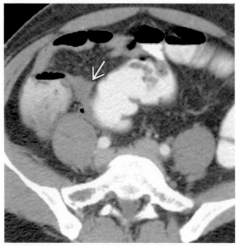

Same patient as previous page. A small amount of free fluid is noted (arrow). Such free fluid, when located between leaves of mesentery, may form an acute angle; such a configuration is rarely seen with fluid filled bowel.

- o Extravasation of bowel contrast material
- o Fat stranding

Imaging Recommendations
- Triple contrast CT scanning is needed to evaluate possible colon injury: Intravenous, oral and colonic contrast material
  - o Colon contrast allows evaluation of the colonic wall and may show extravasation, neither of which is reliable with only oral contrast
- Technique to evaluate colon injury from penetrating or blunt trauma
  - o Colon contrast: 40 mL iodinated contrast in 1,000 mL bag of saline; connect with IV tubing to pediatric rectal catheter; fill to tolerance or by gravity with bag at three feet above table
  - o Scanner and IV contrast: 5 mm thick images and 5 mm image spacing, using an injection rate of at least 2.5 mL/sec for 135-180 mL of contrast, and using a 75 sec delay after beginning injection until starting the scan at the dome of the diaphragm
  - o CT should include both the abdomen and pelvis regardless of site of impact of blunt or penetrating trauma

Differential Diagnosis
- None relevant to this case

Pathology
- None relevant to this case

Clinical Issues
Presentation
- No specific signs or symptoms of colon injury; tenderness, rigidity and absence of bowel sounds may be found
- If injury is retroperitoneal, clinical findings may be delayed

Natural History
- Infection with peritonitis or abscess may occur if there is extraluminal

Treatment

- Surgery is usually undertaken if there are findings of colon injury
- As shown in the figures, perforation may have occurred without free air or extravasation of contrast

Selected References

1. Weishaupt D et al: Traumatic injuries: Imaging of abdominal and pelvic injuries. Eur Radiol. 12:1295-311, 2002
2. Killeen KL et al: Helical computed tomography of bowel and mesenteric injuries. J Trauma. 51:26-36, 2001
3. Shanmuganathan K et al: Triple-contrast helical CT in penetrating torso trauma: A prospective study to determine peritoneal violation and the need for laparotomy. AJR Am J Roentgenol. 177:1247-56, 2001

Mesenteric Injury

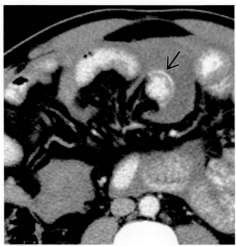

Contrast is seen flowing around a small bowel loop (arrow). The contrast could have come from within bowel or represent active arterial bleeding. The walls of the small bowel appeared normal. At surgery a bleeding mesenteric artery was found.

Key Facts
- Definition: Mesenteric edema, hematoma or active bleeding may be present with mesenteric injury
- Other key facts
  - Accuracy of CT in diagnosing mesenteric injury has not been established by large series
    - False negative diagnoses infrequent
    - Predicting the need for surgery with CT possible in about 75% of mesenteric injuries
  - Surgery needed if active bleeding or hematoma surrounding bowel is seen at CT
  - Mesenteric injury frequently seen with bowel injury

Imaging Findings
General Features
- Best imaging clue: Active mesenteric bleeding or mesenteric hematoma

CT Findings
- Fat stranding within mesenteric fat
- Focal soft tissue density with mesentery – hematoma
- Extravasation of contrast from mesenteric artery

Imaging Recommendations
- CT is the imaging modality of choice
- US may detect free fluid in the unstable patient but the false negative rate with US is about 40% for bowel and mesenteric injuries
- CT technique includes oral and intravenous contrast with 5 mm thick images and 5 mm image spacing, using an injection rate of at least 2.5 mL/sec for 135-180 mL of contrast, and using a 75 sec delay after beginning injection until starting the scan at the dome of the diaphragm
- CT should include both the abdomen and pelvis

Mesenteric Injury

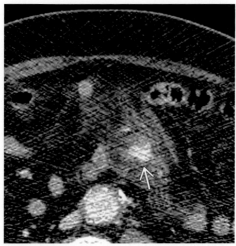

Density consistent with extravasation of arterial contrast is seen in mid abdomen (arrow) with surrounding hematoma. At surgery a mesenteric hematoma was found.

Differential Diagnosis
Mesenteric Edema
- Diffuse fat stranding may be seen especially in the small bowel mesentery with
  - Rapid fluid replacement
  - "Shock bowel"

Pathology
- None relevant to this case

Clinical Issues
Presentation
- Clinical findings in patients with mesenteric injury are non-specific and include abdominal tenderness and possibly hypotension

Treatment
- Surgery necessary with evidence of active arterial extravasation or hematoma which appears to surround bowel loops

Prognosis
- Poor outcome usually the result of associated injuries

Selected References
1. Hanks PW et al: Blunt injury to mesentery and small bowel: CT evaluation. Radiol Clin North Am. 41:1171-82, 2003
2. Hawkins AE et al: Evaluation of bowel and mesenteric injury: Role of multidetector CT. Abdom Imaging. 28:505-14, 2003
3. Killeen KL et al: Helical computed tomography of bowel and mesenteric injuries. J Trauma. 51:26-36, 2001

Duodenal Injury

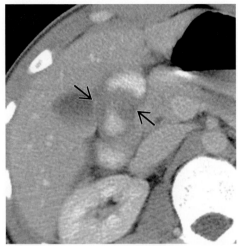

Axial CT scan shows thickening of the wall of the second portion of the duodenum (arrows). In the setting of blunt trauma, hematoma of the duodenal wall would be the diagnosis.

Key Facts
- Definition: Hematoma or perforation of duodenum
- Classic imaging appearance: Thickening of the duodenal wall; presence of retroperitoneal free air
- Other key facts
  - Duodenal injury is seen is about 8% of gastrointestinal tract injuries due to blunt trauma
  - Associated injuries, especially of the pancreas, are frequent
  - Perforation occurs in about 20% of duodenal injuries
    - CT will detect about 60% of perforations of the duodenum

Imaging Findings
General Features
- Best imaging clue: Hematoma of the duodenal wall
- Anatomy
  - Much of the duodenum is retroperitoneal and free air usually would be retroperitoneal rather than intraperitoneal

CT Findings
- Duodenal abnormalities
  - Duodenal wall thickening
  - Wall enhancement
- Paraduodenal abnormalities
  - Free retroperitoneal fluid
  - Free retroperitoneal air
  - Extravasation of oral contrast
  - Fat stranding

Imaging Recommendations
- To maximize sensitivity of CT, oral and intravenous contrast should be used

Duodenal Injury

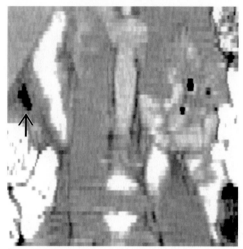

Coronally reformatted CT scan shows both thickening of the duodenal wall and free retroperitoneal air (arrow). As is usually the case, there was not extravasation of oral contrast. The presence of oral contrast, however, allows detection of the bowel wall thickening.

- Duodenal injury is detected on contrast enhanced CT using 5 mm thick images and 5 mm image spacing, using an injection rate of at least 2.5 mL/sec for 135-180 mL of contrast in adults, and using a 75 sec delay after beginning injection until starting the scan at the dome of the diaphragm

Differential Diagnosis
- None relevant to this case

Pathology
- None relevant to this case

Clinical Issues
Presentation
- Duodenal injury has no specific acute findings
- Upper abdominal wall bruising and tenderness may be seen
- Duodenal obstruction due to hematoma may result in vomiting
Treatment
- Duodenal wall hematoma may be treated conservatively; perforation usually requires surgery, although there are case reports of successful nonoperative management of duodenal rupture

Selected References
1. Desai KM et al: Blunt duodenal injuries in children. J Trauma. 54:645-6, 2003
2. Hughes TM et al: Intra-abdominal gastrointestinal tract injuries following blunt trauma: The experience of an Australian trauma centre. Injury. 33:617-26, 2002
3. Soeta N et al: Successful healing of a blunt duodenal rupture by nonoperative management. J Trauma. 52:979-81, 2002

Pancreatic Injury

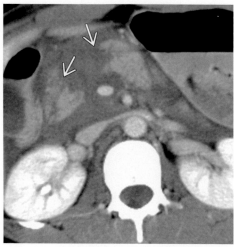

Pancreatic transection is noted with separation of the pancreatic head from the body (arrows). Blood fills the space between the head and body. Blood is also noted in the anterior pararenal space (the retroperitoneal space that is home to the pancreas and duodenum).

Key Facts
- Definition: Laceration or edema of the pancreatic parenchyma after trauma
- Other key facts
  - Pancreatic injury occurs in about 1-3% of patients after blunt trauma
  - 70% of adults and 15-30% of children have associated injuries
    - Liver and duodenum are frequent associated injuries
  - Delay in diagnosis occurs because findings are overlooked or are not visible in the multi-trauma patient
    - Higher mortality occurs if there is delay in diagnosis
    - Sensitivity of CT is less with pancreatic and bowel injury than for other intraabdominal injuries
  - Types of injury
    - Contusion
    - Laceration
    - Fracture
  - Mechanism of injury is thought to be compression of pancreas against the spine due to anterior compression of abdominal wall

Imaging Findings
General Features
- Anatomy: Pancreas resides in the anterior pararenal space
CT Findings
- Contusion or edema is seen as
  - Focal area of lower density within the pancreas
  - Focal area in which there is effacement of the pancreatic septations
- Laceration is seen as a discontinuity in part of the parenchyma

Pancreatic Injury

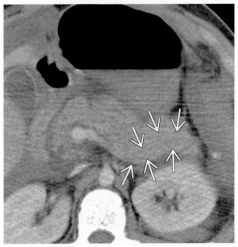

Pancreatic contusion is seen as effacement of the septations in a focal area of the inferior portion of the body of the pancreas (arrows). Septations may not be present, especially in young patients, but if present tend to be uniformly distributed.

- Transection is seen as a laceration across the entire width of the pancreas
- Duct injury is not a CT diagnosis but may be suspected if a laceration extends to the duct and is almost certain in transection
- Secondary findings of injury include
  - Blood in the anterior pararenal space
    - Look for blood between the pancreas and splenic vein, which is normally apposed to the inferior surface of the pancreas
    - Blood may surround the superior mesenteric artery (SMA) and superior mesenteric vein (SMV)/portal vein
  - Fat stranding in the anterior pararenal space
  - Thickening of the left anterior renal fascia

Imaging Recommendations
- Pancreatic injury is detected on contrast enhanced CT using 5 mm thick images and 5 mm image spacing, using an injection rate of at least 2.5 mL/sec for 135-180 mL of contrast, and using a 75 sec delay after beginning injection until starting the scan at the dome of the diaphragm
- If injury is uncertain due to only secondary findings, it may be useful to rescan using thinner sections or reformat to thinner image thickness and spacing
- Duct injury, which occurs in about 15% of patients with pancreatic injury, is not diagnosed with CT but may be demonstrated by ERCP (endoscopic retrograde cholangiopancreatography) or MRI

Differential Diagnosis
- None relevant to this case

Pathology
Staging or Grading Criteria
- American Association for the Surgery of Trauma (AAST)

Pancreatic Injury

- o Type 1: Minor contusion, superficial laceration, duct intact
- o Type 2: Major contusion, major laceration, duct intact
- o Type 3: Duct injury, distal transection
- o Type 4: Proximal transection, ampulla injury
- o Type 5: Massive disruption of pancreatic head
- Lucas Classification
  - o Type 1: Contusion
  - o Type 2: Transection anterior to spine
  - o Type 3: Laceration of pancreatic head
  - o Type 4: Injury of head and duodenum

Clinical Issues
Presentation
- Amylase may initially be normal or abnormal
  - o A normal amylase does not exclude pancreatic injury
  - o An abnormal amylase does not necessarily indicate pancreatic injury
- 1-2 days after injury, the amylase will be elevated in 80-90% of patients with pancreatic injury

Natural History
- Weeks to years later the following may occur
  - o Recurrent pancreatitis
  - o Pancreatic abscess
  - o Hemorrhage
  - o Pseudocyst(s)
  - o Fistulae to adjacent structures
  - o Duct stricture

Treatment
- Injury to the pancreatic duct constitutes a surgical emergency

Selected References
1. Ilahi O et al: Efficacy of computed tomography in the diagnosis of pancreatic injury in adult blunt trauma patients: A single-institutional study. Am Surg. 68:704-7, 2002
2. Patch SV et al: Imaging of pancreatic trauma. Br J Radiol 71:985-90, 1998
3. Lucas CE: Diagnosis and treatment of pancreatic and duodenal injury. Surg Clin North Am. 57:49-65, 1977

Renal Parenchymal Trauma

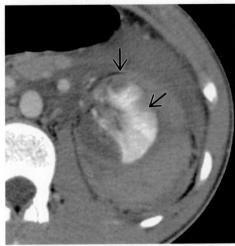

Axial CT image shows a large amount of blood in the perirenal space. In addition there are wedge shaped areas of hypoperfusion of the renal parenchyma (arrows). The wedge shape suggests damage to arterial branches and areas of infarct.

Key Facts
- Renal trauma is the most common retroperitoneal injury
  - About 10% of injuries from blunt abdominal trauma involve the kidney
- Types of injury of renal parenchyma
  - Contusion
  - Subcapsular hematoma
  - Laceration
  - Fractured kidney
  - Shattered kidney
  - Intraparenchymal vascular injury
  - Intraparenchymal collecting system injury
- Urinoma may be delayed hours to days after an initial scan

Imaging Findings
General Features
- Best imaging clue: Abnormality of the nephrogram and blood adjacent to parenchyma
- Anatomy
  - Perirenal space may connect with the pararenal spaces
  - Perirenal space continues inferiorly anterior to the psoas around the ureter
CT Findings
- Contusion: Striations noted in the parenchymal arterial phase
- Subcapsular hematoma: Blood density collection which compresses the parenchyma around a portion of the kidney circumference
- Laceration: Linear area of hypoperfusion in the parenchyma extending partially through the kidney
- Fracture: Laceration which goes through the parenchyma separating the kidney into at least two fragments
- Shattered kidney: Multiple fractures

Renal Parenchymal Trauma

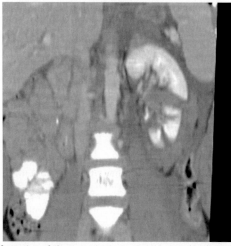

Coronal reformation of the same patient as previous page shows the multiple fractures crossing the parenchyma characteristic of a shattered kidney. Blood is seen separating the renal fragments.

- Intraparenchymal vascular injury: Traumatic arterial occlusion leading to hypoperfusion of a portion of the kidney
- Intraparenchymal collecting system injury: Tear of calyces, infundibula or real pelvis allowing extravasation of urine into the perirenal space

Imaging Recommendations
- Renal trauma is best depicted at CT using 5 mm thick images and 5 mm image spacing, using an injection rate of at least 2.5 mL/sec for 135-180 mL of contrast, and using a 75 sec delay after beginning injection until starting the scan at the dome of the diaphragm
- Scanning is delayed at the iliac crest in any abdominal trauma CT and then extended into the pelvis, which should allow opacification of the distal ureters
- Delayed scanning or repeat scan may demonstrate expanding hematoma or extravasation of opacified urine

Differential Diagnosis
- None relevant to this case

Pathology
Staging or Grading Criteria of Renal Injury
- Grade I
  - No laceration
  - Contusion
  - Non-expanding subcapsular hematoma
- Grade II
  - Laceration < 1 cm long
  - Non-expanding hematoma
- Grade III
  - Laceration > 1 cm
  - No urinary extravasation

- Grade IV
  - o Fractured kidney extending through the collecting system
  - o Vascular hemorrhage
- Grade V
  - o Shattered kidney
  - o Avulsion of renal hilum with devascularized kidney

Clinical Issues

Presentation
- Gross hematuria
- Microscopic hematuria
- Hypotension

Natural History
- Pressure within the retroperitoneum will tend to tamponade injuries resulting in conservative management of even severe injuries

Treatment
- Stent placement is needed to decompress the collecting system if there is urine extravasation; foley catheter placement decompresses the bladder
- Embolization may be needed for continued bleeding
  - o Control of bleeding is successful in about 90% with embolization
- Nephrectomy may be needed with uncontrolled bleeding

Prognosis
- Complications following non-operative management include
  - o Continued hemorrhage
  - o Pseudoaneurysm
  - o Artrio-venous fistula
  - o Hypertension, which may be transient
  - o Renal failure
  - o Urinoma, which may become infected
  - o Abscess

Selected References
1. Harris AC et al: CT findings in blunt renal trauma. Radiographics. 21:S201-14, 2001
2. Santucci RA et al: Grade IV renal injuries: Evaluation, treatment, and outcome. World J Surg. 25:1565-72, 2001
3. Mirvis SE et al: Trauma. Advances in Uroradiology. Radiol Clin North Am. 34:1225-57, 1996

Renal Pedicle Injury

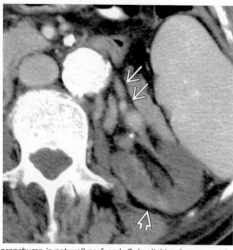

The renal parenchyma is not well perfused. Only slight enhancement is seen infero-medially (open arrow) due to supply from the capsular arteries. There is contrast in the renal artery near its takeoff from the aorta (arrows).

Key Facts
- Definition: Vascular pedicle injuries include laceration or avulsion of the renal artery or vein and thrombosis of renal artery or vein
  - Renal pedicle also includes the uretero-pevic junction
- Classic imaging appearance
  - Arterial thrombosis – lack of perfusion of kidney
  - Venous thrombosis – prolonged nephrogram
- Other key facts
  - Renal pedicle injury indicator of high energy trauma, thus associated spine or intraabdominal injuries very frequent
  - Vascular pedicle injuries occur in < 5% of injuries to the kidney
    - Injury may be due to blunt or penetrating trauma
    - In blunt trauma injury results from stretching or shearing forces on the renal pedicle

Imaging Findings
General Features
- Best imaging clue
  - Arterial injury: Nonenhancement of kidney
  - Venous injury: Asymmetric prolonged density on the side of injury
- Anatomy: Kidneys, aorta and IVC are in the perirenal space
CT Findings
- NECT: Vascular thrombosis may appear hyperdense relative to unenhanced blood
- CECT
  - Laceration
    - Large retroperitoneal (perirenal space) hematoma; active bleeding may be seen around kidney, aorta and IVC
  - Arterial thrombosis
    - Abrupt lack of opacification of renal artery beginning at thrombosis

Renal Pedicle Injury

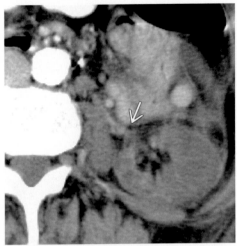

The obstruction to flow of contrast in the renal artery is seen (arrow). This is most likely due to intimal tear and thrombosis. There is slight enhancement at the periphery of the kidney, the result of patent capsular blood supply.

- Absence of nephrogram and excretion
- Peripheral (rim) enhancement of kidney from capsular arteries
- Normal sized kidney
  - o Venous thrombosis (rare)
    - Decreased early nephrogram
    - Prolonged nephrogram
    - Decreased or absent excretion of contrast
    - Enlarged kidney and renal vein
    - Filling defect, thrombus, within vein
    - Delayed appearance of peripheral enhancement

Imaging Recommendations
- Renal pedicle injury should prompt obtaining a follow-up scan to look for urinoma or expanding hematoma

Differential Diagnosis
- None relevant to this case

Pathology
- None relevant to this case

Clinical Issues
Treatment
- Active bleeding and expanding hematoma increase the likelihood of surgery

Prognosis
- Arterial or venous thrombosis may lead to renal infarction
- Delayed systemic hypertension may develop due to renal ischemia (Page kidney)
- Other complications

Renal Pedicle Injury

- Abscess
- Urinoma
- Artero-venous fistula

Selected References
1. Kawashima A et al: Imaging evaluation of posttraumatic renal injuries. Abdom Imaging. 27:199-213, 2002
2. Sclafani SJ et al: CT diagnosis of renal pedicle injury. Urol Radiol. 7:63-8, 1985
3. Steinberg DL et al: The computerized tomography appearance of renal pedicle injury. J Urol. 132:1163-4, 1984

Traumatic Urinoma

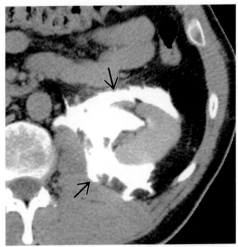

A traumatic urinoma is seen because of extravasation of contrast-laden urine into the perirenal space. The contrast partially surrounds the kidney and obscures the renal pelvis. These delayed images were obtained because of perirenal fluid seen on the initial CT scan.

Key Facts
- Definition: Extravasation of urine from a traumatic tear in the renal collecting system or ureter
- Other key facts
  - Results from trauma of intrerenal collecting system, renal pelvis or ureter
  - Most common ureteral injury is avulsion at uretero-pelvic junction, most commonly in children or adolescents
  - On initial trauma CT, traumatic urinoma may be suspected because of fluid (unopacificated urine) in the perirenal space, which may dissect down anterior to the psoas
    - Diagnosis frequently made on delayed images which reveal extravasation of urine and excreted contrast material
  - Mechanism
    - Compression of kidney or ureter against lumbar spine
    - Deceleration injury with tearing near the renal pelvis
  - Hematuria may be absent
    - In about 30% of ureteral injuries, hematuria is absent

Imaging Findings
General Features
- Best imaging clue: High density contrast material in perirenal space on delayed images
- Anatomy
  - The perirenal space surrounds the kidneys, aorta, and IVC and extends inferiorly around the ureter anterior to the psoas muscle
- CT Findings

Traumatic Urinoma

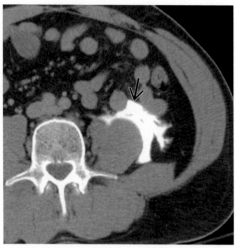

Excreted contrast in the same patient as previous page dissects inferiorly just anterior to the psoas muscle within the inferior extension of the perirenal space, which continues down around the ureter.

- o On arterial phase trauma CT low density (10 HU) fluid, unopacified urine, may be seen in the perirenal space; may be higher density if mixed with blood
- o During arterial phase of trauma CT high density contrast extravasation would be of arterial origin
- o During the renal excretory phase, seen on delayed images, high density contrast extravasation will be from the ureter, renal pelvis, or intrarenal collecting system
- o If questionable findings, delay should be extended to 10-15 minutes
- o Renal nephrogram and excretion will occur with expected timing and will be symmetric if vascular injury has not occurred
- o The distal ureter may not opacify with contrast material in avulsion at UVJ or in ureteral transection

Imaging Recommendations
- Abdominal and pelvic trauma CT performed with oral and intravenous contrast enhanced CT using 5 mm thick images and 5 mm image spacing, using an injection rate of at least 2.5 mL/sec for 135-180 mL of contrast, and using a 75 sec delay after beginning injection until starting the scan at the dome of the diaphragm and ending below the ischial tuberosities
- Fluid in the perirenal space should prompt delayed images during the renal excretory phase

Differential Diagnosis
Non-Traumatic Urinoma
- Urinoma may occur due to obstruction of the ureter with rupture of the intrarenal collecting system at the fornix of a calyx
  - o Such obstruction may be due to blood clot, stone, tumor, congenital obstruction in children, retroperitoneal fibrosis and iatrogenic causes

Traumatic Urinoma

Pathology
- None relevant to this case

Clinical Issues
Presentation
- Hematuria may be seen with injury to the renal collecting system or ureter; this is neither sensitive nor specific for presence of urinoma
- Flank tenderness
- Lumbar spine transverse process fractures may be noted

Treatment
- If the ureter is not avulsed, a stent from the urinary bladder to the renal pelvis will decompress the collecting system and allow a ureteral tear to heal
- Avulsion at the uretero-pelvic junction or ureteral transection would be treated surgically

Prognosis
- Healing usually occurs without adverse sequelae
- Urinoma may become infected leading to abscess
- Delayed retroperitoneal fibrosis could lead to ureteral obstruction

Selected References
1. Novelline RA et al: Helical CT of abdominal trauma. Radiol Clin North Am. 37:591- 612, 1999
2. Toporoff B et al: Ureteral laceration caused by a fall from a height: Case report and review of the literature. J Trauma. 34:164-4, 1993
3. Titton RL et al: Urine leaks and urinomas: Diagnosis and imaging-guided intervention. Radiographics. 23(5):1133-47, 2003

Adrenal Injury

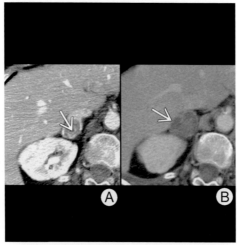

(A) CT scan immediately following trauma shows active hemorrhage (arrow) into the adrenal, which appears enlarged. (B) Two weeks later the mass due to hemorrhage (arrow) is still seen and appears somewhat larger than on the initial scan.

Key Facts
- Definition: Adrenal injury is seen as an abnormality of size or shape of the adrenal
- Other key facts
  - Adrenal injury is seen in about 2% of patients with blunt trauma
  - Associated injuries occur in 90% of patients
  - Injury is usually unilateral, right side more frequent than left

Imaging Findings
General Features
- Anatomy: The adrenal glands are located in the perirenal space with the kidneys, aorta and inferior vena cava
CT Findings
- Abnormalities of the adrenal
  - Round or oval mass is seen (80%)
  - Diffuse hemorrhage may obscure the adrenal (10%)
  - Adrenal may appear uniformly enlarged and indistinct (10%)
- Abnormalities adjacent to the adrenal
  - Hemorrhage
  - Fat stranding
  - Thickening of adjacent fascia
  - Thickening of diaphragmatic crus
Imaging Recommendations
- Adrenal injury is detected on contrast enhanced CT using 5 mm thick images and 5 mm image spacing, using an injection rate of at least 2.5 mL/sec for 135-180 mL of contrast, and using a 75 sec delay after beginning injection until starting the scan at the dome of the diaphragm
- If the only finding at CT is a hemorrhage in the shape of a mass, follow-up CT or MRI should be performed to exclude adrenal neoplasm

Adrenal Injury

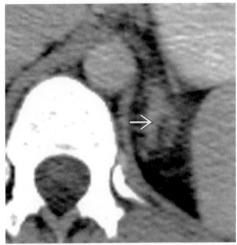

The left adrenal gland appeared indistinct at CT with slight adjacent fat stranding. The discharge diagnosis included adrenal injury as a result (arrow).

- A hematoma should resolve by 6 months
- The adrenal gland may atrophy by 12 months

Differential Diagnosis
Adrenal Neoplasm

Pathology
- None relevant to this case

Clinical Issues
Natural History
- An adrenal hematoma will decrease in size and attenuation over time
Prognosis
- Bilateral adrenal injury may lead to acute adrenal crisis
  - Hypokalemia
  - Hyponatremia
  - Hypotension
  - Acidosis

Selected References
1. Oto A et al: Delayed posttraumatic adrenal hematoma. Eur Radiol. 10:903-5, 2000
2. Novelline RA et al: Extraperitoneal abdominal injuries. Radiol Clin North Am. 37:591-612, 1999
3. Burks DW et al: Acute adrenal injury after blunt abdominal trauma: CT findings. AJR Am J Roentgenol. 158:503-7, 1992

Inferior Vena Cava Injury

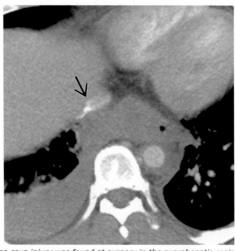

Inferior vena cava injury was found at surgery in the suprahepatic region. Note the irregular contour of the IVC (arrow) and surrounding blood. There is also blood in the mediastinum and a right hemothorax.

Key Facts
- Definition: Tear or rupture of the IVC
- Classic imaging appearance: Pericaval hematoma and irregular caval contour
  - Contrast extravasation may not be seen due to low pressure in cava and tamponade effect of adjacent hematoma
- Other key facts
  - Surgery is progressively more difficult depending on location of IVC injury
    - Mortality with retrohepatic IVC injury and associated injuries exceeds 50%
  - IVC injuries account for 30-40% of major abdominal vascular injuries
    - Most from penetrating trauma

Imaging Findings
General Features
- Anatomy
  - Location of IVC
    - Infrarenal
    - Suprarenal and infrahepatic
    - Retrohepatic or suprahepatic
CT Findings
- Irregularity of IVC contour
- Indistinct edge of IVC
- Narrowing of lumen
- Abrupt cutoff
- Contrast extravasation
- Hemorrhage with IVC at epicenter
- Contained hematoma (pseudoaneurysm) of IVC - rare
- Liver laceration extending to porta or IVC

Inferior Vena Cava Injury

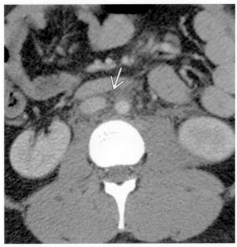

Blood around the IVC and aorta (arrow) in the same patient as above is noted in the infrahepatic region. This blood may have dissected down from the suprahepatic tear since no other injury was found in the perirenal space.

- Intraluminal fat in IVC – rare
- IVC thrombosis – rare - delayed appearance days to years after injury

Imaging Recommendations
- Trauma CT is imaging procedure of choice: 5 mm thick images and spacing, 15 mm/sec table speed, e.g., 4 x 2.5 mm detector configuration, intravenous and oral contrast administration

Differential Diagnosis
Hypotension
- Flattened IVC over a long segment is a characteristic of hypovolemia
  - o Injured IVC may appear slit-like at the injured segment

Hematoma Adjacent to IVC
- Hemorrhage from another source may surround the IVC in the perirenal space or retrohepatic area

Pathology
- None relevant to this case

Clinical Issues
Presentation
- History of major trauma
- Possible hypotension and tachycardia
- No specific signs or symptoms of IVC injury

Treatment
- Instability of patient or findings suspicious for IVC injury results in surgical exploration

Prognosis
- Depends of associated injuries
- Depends on location of IVC injury
  - o Poor prognosis with retrohepatic or suprahepatic injury

Inferior Vena Cava Injury

Selected References
1. Hewett JJ et al: The spectrum of abdominal venous CT findings in blunt trauma. AJR Am J Roentgenol. 176:955-8, 2001
2. Hewett JJ et al: Contained hematoma (pseudoaneurysm) of the inferior vena cava associated with blunt abdominal trauma. AJR Am J Roentgenol. 172:1144, 1999
3. Kimoto T et al: Inferior vena cava thrombosis after traumatic liver injury. HPB Surg. 11:111-6, 1998

Abdominal Aorta Injury

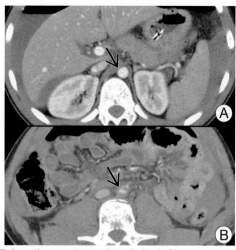

(A) Axial CT shows the normal aorta above the level of injury (arrow). (B) Axial CT at a lower level shows irregularity of the aortic contour with narrowing of the lumen (arrow).

Key Facts
- Injury of the abdominal aorta is rare
- 70% of patients have associated injuries, especially spine fractures and bowel injury as seen in the "seat belt syndrome"
- Location of injury is most frequent just below the renal arteries
- Types of abdominal aortic injury
  - Thrombosis or occlusion, intramural hematoma, acute pseudoaneurysm or late true aneurysm, aortic rupture or disruption, localized intimal injury may lead to isolated abdominal aortic dissection or thrombosis

Imaging Findings
General Features
- Best imaging clue: Narrowing of aortic lumen at CT
- Other generic features
  - Location near inferior mesenteric artery (IMA) felt due to lap belt compressing aorta against spine in MVC and may be termed "seat belt aorta"
CT Findings
- Thrombosis may be partial or complete
  - Narrowing of lumen of aorta is seen
- Rupture leads to periaortic hematoma if patient survives to imaging
- Intramural hematoma may be difficult to detect because of contrast in the lumen at trauma abdominal CT
Imaging Recommendations
- Aortic injury is best detected on contrast enhanced CT using 5 mm thick images and 5 mm image spacing, using an injection rate of at least 2.5 mL/sec for 135-180 mL of contrast, and using a 75 sec delay after beginning injection until starting scan at the dome of diaphragm

Abdominal Aorta Injury

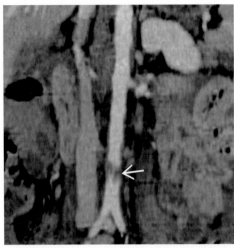

Curved plane CT reformation from axial CT data shows the abdominal aorta with initial tear and focus of thrombus narrowing the lumen (arrow). Reformation depicts the extent of the injury. Patient had a stent placed with good recovery.

- Scanning should include both abdomen & pelvis Sagittal, coronal & curved plane reformations viewing with soft tissue window will display nature & extent of injury

Differential Diagnosis
- None relevant to this case

Pathology
- None relevant to this case

Clinical Issues
Presentation
- With sufficient obstruction to arterial flow, the patient may have decreased or absent femoral pulses
- Injury to aorta may lead to hypotension if has been extensive bleeding
- Rupture may lead to death before CT can be obtained
Treatment
- Stent placement if there is no rupture
- Emergency surgery may be needed if there is evidence of extraluminal blood
Prognosis
- Depends on the severity of the injury
  o Treated thrombosis may result in total recovery
  o Rupture may lead to death

Selected References
1. Inaba K et al: Blunt abdominal aortic trauma in association with thoracolumbar spine fractures. Injury. 32:201-7, 2001
2. Marty-Ane CH et al: Intravascular stenting of traumatic abdominal aortic dissection. J Vasc Surg. 23:156-61, 1996
3. Lock JS et al: Blunt trauma to the abdominal aorta. J Trauma. 27:674-7, 1987

Traumatic Lumbar Rupture

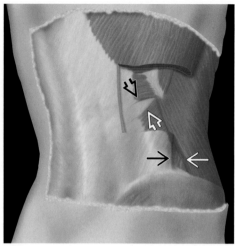

Drawing shows the borders of the inferior (arrows) and superior (open arrows) lumbar triangles.

Key Facts

- Definition: Herniation of fat and/or bowel through the abdominal wall at the superior or inferior lumbar triangles
- Classic imaging appearance: Bulging or herniation of intraabdominal fat or bowel through defect in the postero-lateral abdominal wall
- Other key facts
  - Traumatic lumbar hernia is rare but more frequent than other traumatic abdominal wall hernias such as inguinal or Spigelian
  - Mechanism
    - Shear stress associated with acute elevation of intraabdominal pressure
    - In addition to trauma, cause may be infection, prior surgical site or spontaneous
  - Seat belt use related to this injury if rotation and flexion of the body occur
  - Presentation may be delayed days or months
  - Associated injuries (over 30% of patients with abdominal wall hernias) include bowel and mesentery, diaphragm, solid viscera, bladder and fractures of spine and pelvis

Imaging Findings

General Features

- Anatomy of the two lumbar triangles
- Superior lumbar triangle: Triangle of Grynfelt described in 1866
  - 12th rib superiorly
  - Internal oblique muscle laterally
  - Quadratus lumborum muscle medially
- Inferior lumbar triangle: Petit's triangle described in 1774
  - Iliac crest inferiorly
  - External oblique muscle anteriorly
  - Latissimus dorsi muscle posteriorly

Traumatic Lumbar Rupture

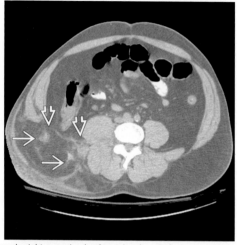

Hernia through right superior lumbar triangle. Defect seen in aponeurosis of transversalis muscle (open arrows). Intraabdominal fat has herniated through the defect and there is stranding in the fat. Within the fat, areas of blood are seen (arrows).

<u>CT Findings</u>
- Posterolateral defect in abdominal wall muscle or fascia
  - Defect in superficial surface of superior triangle: Latissimus dorsi
  - Defect in deep surface of superior triangle: Aponeurosis of transversalis
  - Defect in superficial surface of inferior triangle: Superficial fascia
  - Defect in deep surface of inferior triangle: Internal oblique
- Muscles from side to side will appear asymmetric
- Content of hernia
  - Intraperitoneal fat
  - Small bowel or colon

<u>Imaging Recommendations</u>
- Trauma protocol for abdominal and pelvic CT using intravenous and oral contrast includes, for example, 5 mm thick image and spacing, 15 mm/sec table speed and detector configuration of 4 x 5 mm
- Even if lumbar hernia is evident clinically and definition of the hernia defect could be made without contrast, contrast would be indicated because of associated injuries

Differential Diagnosis
- None relevant to this case

Pathology
- None relevant to this case

Clinical Issues
<u>Presentation</u>
- Flank ecchymosis or hematoma or bulging
- Localized flank pain or referred pain to anterior abdominal wall or sciatic distribution

Traumatic Lumbar Rupture

- "Seat belt sign", bruising of anterior abdominal wall from seat belt compression

Treatment
- Laparotomy because of associated injury and risk of incarceration or strangulation of bowel
- Endoscopic repair has been reported

Prognosis
- With bowel displacement into hernia, incarceration will occur in about 25% and strangulation in 10% of patients
- Other complications include bowel contusion, bowel ischemia from mesenteric vascular tear and bowel obstruction of small bowel or colon

Selected References
1. Guillem P et al: Lumbar hernia: Anatomical route assessed by computed tomography. Surg Radiol Anat. 24:53-6, 2002
2. Hickey MB et al: Computed tomography of traumatic abdominal wall hernia and associated deceleration injuries. Can Assoc radiol J. 53:153-9, 2002
3. Lee GH et al: CT imaging of abdominal hernias. AJR Am J Roentgenol. 161:1209-13, 1993

Extraperitoneal Bladder Injury

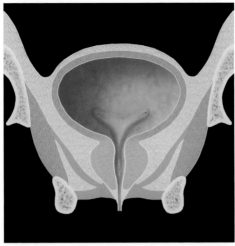

Drawing shows the fat surrounding the bladder. The space in which the fat is located extends anteriorly along the abdominal wall to the level of the umbilicus. This fat extends laterally to the iliac vessels and to the presacral space and extends inferiorly to the inguinal canals.

Key Facts
- Definition: In extraperitoneal bladder injury the bladder wall may be contused and intact or the bladder wall may rupture into the extraperitoneal spaces continuous with the bladder
- Other key facts
  - Extraperitoneal rupture is the most frequent location of urinary bladder rupture occurring in 80+% of patients with bladder ruptures
  - Diagnosis with CT is very accurate with sensitivity and specificity of nearly 100%
  - Mechanism is either
    - Blunt trauma causing increased pressure within the bladder and rupture
    - Penetration of the bladder by a fracture fragment or foreign body
  - Associated injuries of other organs or bony structures are seen in over 90% of patients with bladder rupture

Imaging Findings
General Features
- Best imaging clue: At CT low density (about 10 HU) fluid in the extraperitoneal spaces or bladder contrast extravasating into the extraperitoneal spaces will be seen, which does not surround bowel loops
- Other generic features: Bladder contrast extravasating into the anterior abdominal wall (anterior prevesicle space) or along the lateral abdominal wall or pelvic side walls may cause misdiagnosis of intraperitoneal injury
- Anatomy: Extraperitoneal spaces into which bladder rupture extends include

Extraperitoneal Bladder Injury

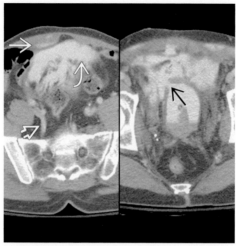

(A) Superior to the bladder the extravasation of bladder of contrast is seen in the anterior prevesicle space (arrow), the perivesical space (curved arrow) and the pelvic sidewall (open arrow). (B) The point of rupture of the bladder wall with extravasating contrast can be seen (arrow).

- o Anterior prevesicle space, presacral space, perivesicle space, perineum
- o Thigh

CT Findings
- There may not be bladder contrast extravasation unless there is sufficient pressure in the bladder
- Urine will appear as low density (5-10 HU) fluid and bladder contrast as very high density fluid in the extraperitoneal spaces as described above

Imaging Recommendations
- CT cystogram is required so that a known volume of contrast creates sufficient pressure to cause extravasation; a "full appearing bladder" at trauma CT does not exclude rupture
- CT cystogram is indicated with hematuria, pelvic fractures, or low density fluid in the intraperitoneal or extraperitoneal spaces
- CT cystogram technique
  - o Unclamp Foley and drain bladder
  - o Instill 400-500 mL 4% iodinated contrast (pressure of 40 cm water)
  - o Repeat pelvic CT images

Differential Diagnosis
Intraperitoneal Bladder Rupture
- Intraperitoneal urine or contrast will be within the intraperitoneal spaces and frequently will appear to surround bowel loops

Combined Intraperitoneal and Extraperitoneal Bladder Rupture
- Occurs in 5-10% of patients with bladder rupture

Pathology
- None relevant to this case

Extraperitoneal Bladder Injury

Clinical Issues

Presentation

- 70-100% of patients who have bladder rupture will have gross hematuria

Treatment

- Extraperitoneal bladder rupture is treated only with decompression with a Foley catheter
  - Intraperitoneal rupture will cause electrolyte problems if treated conservatively and surgery is required

Selected References
1. Deck AJ et al: Current experience with computed tomography cystography and blunt trauma. World J Surg. 25:1592-6, 2001
2. Morey AF et al: Bladder rupture after blunt trauma: Guidelines for diagnostic imaging. J Trauma. 51:683-6, 2001
3. Morgan DE et al: CT cystography: Radiographic and clinical predictors of bladder rupture. AJR am J Roentgenol. 174:89-95, 2000

Intraperitoneal Bladder Injury

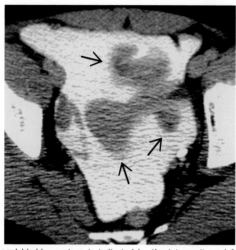

Intraperitoneal bladder rupture is indicated by the intraperitoneal free contrast surrounding bowel loops (arrows).

Key Facts
- Definition: With intraperitoneal bladder rupture the bladder wall is torn and there is rupture of urine into the intraperitoneal spaces
- Other key facts
  - Intraperitoneal rupture occurs in 10-20% of patients with bladder ruptures
  - Studies have shown that there may be false negative diagnoses specifically for intraperitoneal rupture; to exclude intraperitoneal rupture, CT cystogram is imperative
  - Mechanism is either
    - Blunt trauma causing increased pressure within the bladder and rupture
    - Penetration of the bladder by a fracture fragment or foreign body
  - Associated injuries of other organs or bony structures are seen in over 90% of patients with bladder rupture

Imaging Findings
General Features
- Best imaging clue: CT low density (about 10 HU) fluid or bladder contrast surrounding bowel loops
- Anatomy: Intraperitoneal spaces into which bladder rupture most frequently extends include
  - Perisplenic and perihepatic spaces
  - Morrison's pouch
  - Pericolic gutters
  - Pelvis
CT Findings
- There may not be contrast extravasation unless there is sufficient pressure in the bladder
- Urine will appear as low density (5-10 HU) fluid and bladder contrast as very high density fluid in the intraperitoneal spaces as described above

198

Intraperitoneal Bladder Injury

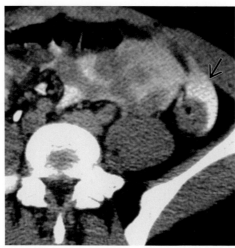

With intraperitoneal bladder rupture contrast may be seen in the paracolic gutters as in this patient (arrow).

Imaging Recommendations
- CT cystogram is required so that a known volume of contrast creates sufficient pressure to cause extravasation; a "full appearing bladder" at trauma CT does not exclude rupture
- CT cystogram is indicated with hematuria, pelvic fractures, or low density fluid in the intraperitoneal or extraperitoneal spaces
  o A few patients will have bladder rupture without hematuria
- CT cystogram technique
  o Unclamp Foley and drain bladder
  o Instill 400-500 mL 4% iodinated contrast (pressure of 40 cm water)
  o Repeat pelvic CT images

Differential Diagnosis
Extraperitoneal Bladder Rupture
- Extra peritoneal urine or contrast will be within the extraperitoneal spaces
  o The anterior prevesicle space extends along the anterior abdominal wall to the level of the umbilicus and contrast may extend laterally adjacent to the properitoneal fat; this can be confused for intraperitoneal extravasation
Combined Intraperitoneal and Extraperitoneal Bladder Rupture
- Occurs in 5-10% of patients with bladder rupture

Pathology
- None relevant to this case

Clinical Issues
Presentation
- 70-100% of patients who have bladder rupture will have gross hematuria

Intraperitoneal Bladder Injury

Treatment
- Intraperitoneal rupture will cause electrolyte problems if treated conservatively and surgery is required
  - Extraperitoneal rupture may be treated with a Foley catheter only

Selected References
1. Hsieh C et al: Diagnosis and management of bladder injury by trauma surgeons. Am J Surg. 184:143-7, 2002
2. Vaccaro JP et al: CT cystography in the evaluation off major bladder trauma. Radiographics. 20:1373-81, 2000
3. Peng MY et al: CT cystography versus conventional cystography in evaluation of bladder injury. AJR Am J Roentgenol. 173:1269-72, 1999

Urethral Injury

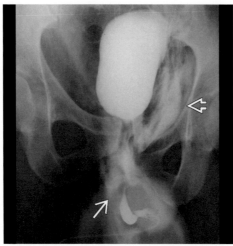

Retrograde urethrogram shows extravasation of contrast into the perivesidal space (open arrow) and into the perineum (arrow). Early extravasation fluoroscopically was near junction of anterior and posterior urethra (urogenital diphagram).

Key Facts
- Definition: Contusion, tear or transection of the urethra
- Classic imaging appearance: Extravasation of contrast material during a retrograde urethrogram (RUG)
- Other key facts
  - Injuries may occur from falls, athletic activities, assaults, motor vehicle collisions, penetrating injuries and traumatic catheterizations
  - Bulbous urethra most commonly injured by compression against the pubic bones, for example from a straddle injury
  - Membranous urethra injured in severe pelvic fractures, especially with widening of the pubic symphysis
    - Posterior urethral injuries seen in about 5-10% of pelvic fractures
  - Simultaneous injuries elsewhere occur in about 50% of patients
  - Urethral injury is rare in women
  - Urethral catheterization may transform a urethral tear into an avulsion of the urethra

Imaging Findings
General Features
- Best imaging clue without intraurethral contrast: Perineal hematoma or periurethral fluid
- Anatomy: Male: From urinary bladder to penile meatus
  - Posterior urethra
    - Prostatic urethra: Extends from bladder through prostate
    - Membranous urethra: Extends from prostate to urogenital diaphragm (UGD), which contains urethral sphincter
  - Anterior urethra
    - Bulbous urethra: Extends from UGD through proximal corpus and ischial cavernosus-bulbospongiosus muscles

Urethral Injury

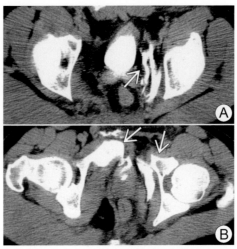

(A) Axial CT of abdomen and pelvis obtained after RUG shows contrast in the perivesical space (arrow). (B) Axial CT shows separation of the pubic symphasis (arrows).

- ▪ Penile urethra: Extends through pendulous portion of penis to the fossa navicularis of the glans
- ○ Female: Urethra 1-2 inches long from urinary bladder to urethral orifice

CT Findings
- Hematoma adjacent to the site of injury
- Contrast extravasation if the base of bladder is involved or if prior RUG has been performed
- Associated injuries such as pelvic fracture and widening of pubic symphysis

MR Findings
- MR can demonstrates urethral disruption, hematoma, length of injury and displacement of apex of prostate

Retrograde Urethrogram Findings
- Type I injury: Prostatic urethra is smoothly narrowed or tapered to a point of relative obstruction due to compression by hematoma
- Type II injury: Extravasation of contrast into the perivesical space above the urogenital diaphragm (UGD) from tear or transection at the prostatic-membranous junction
- Type III: Extravasation into true pelvis and into perineum and possibly into the scrotum from tear or transection involving both anterior and posterior urethra at the UGD
- Type IV: Extravasation into perivesicle space from injury to proximal urethra and bladder neck
- Type V: Extravasation into perineum and scrotum from anterior urethral injury

Imaging Recommendations
- Retrograde urethrogram is performed by placing a small catheter into the fossa navicularis, manually occluding antegrade flow, and injecting under fluoroscopy up to 30 mL of 4% iodinated contrast

- o Injection would be stopped when location of extravasation or point of obstruction to retrograde flow is seen
- CT is needed to assess associated injuries but is not sensitive for urethral injuries

Differential Diagnosis
- None relevant to this case

Pathology
Staging or Grading Criteria
- Type I: No urethral tear or rupture in presence of cephalad displacement of prostate due to disruption of puboprostatic ligaments
  - o Hemorrhage causes narrowing of the prostatic urethra
- Type II: Posterior urethral rupture at prostatic-membranous junction; contrast extravasation into true pelvis
- Type III: Combined anterior and posterior urethral injury at urogenital diaphragm (at membranous urethra) with extravasation into true pelvis and into perineum and possibly into the scrotum
- Type IV: Proximal urethral injury plus injury to bladder neck
- Type V: Anterior urethral injury with extravasation into perineum and possibly into scrotum

Clinical Issues
Presentation
- Bleeding from urethral meatus
- Inability to void
- Pain
- Gross or microscopic hematuria
- Perineal hematoma, ecchymosis
- Pelvic instability
- High-riding or boggy prostate
- Traumatic catheterization
Treatment
- Penetrating trauma: Exploration surgically
- Blunt injury
  - o Tear may be treated by stenting over a urethral catheter and may require surgery, endoscopic repair, or fluoroscopically guided realignment
  - o Transection requires urethroplasty which is best delayed days to weeks but requires urgent suprapubic cystostomy for urinary drainage
  - o Urethral catheter remains after surgery as a stent for duration of healing
Prognosis
- Urethral stenosis may occur, especially if initial injury is not recognized
  - o Recognized by decreased stream and voiding symptoms
  - o Bulbar injuries especially subject to delayed diagnosis

Selected References
1. Ryu J et al: MR imaging of the male and female urethra. Radiographics. 21:1169-85, 2001
2. Boullier JA et al: Early primary endoscopic realignment of posterior urethral injuries. J Urol 151:439A, 1994
3. Munter DW et al: Blunt scrotal trauma: emergency department evaluation and management. Am J Emerg Med. 7:227-34, 1989

Scrotal Trauma

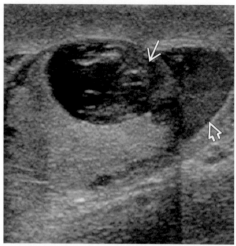

This patient was in a bike accident sustaining scrotal trauma. There appears to be interruption of the tunica albuginea (white arrow) at the edge of an intratesticular hematoma. Also a hematocele (open arrow) with a few internal echoes can be seen.

Key Facts
- Classic imaging appearance: Variation from the almost homogeneous reflectivity or ovoid contour of testis and abnormal fluid collection
- Other key facts
- Variety of injuries to scrotum occur: Soft tissues of scrotum, testis, and epiditymus
  - Testicular injuries: Rupture of tunica albuginea, torsion, dislocation, hematoma, contusion, hematocele
    - Delayed hydrocele or pyocele days to weeks later
    - Right side more frequently injured than left
  - Scrotal soft tissue injuries: Laceration, hematoma
  - Epididymal injuries: Rupture, laceration, hematoma
    - Delayed posttraumatic epididymitis
- Traumatic hydrocele or hematocele is indicative of testicular rupture in over 50% of patients
- Of all testicular torsion, 5-12% are due to trauma
- Associated injury to urethra, bony pelvis

Imaging Findings
<u>General Features</u>
- Anatomy
  - Scrotal midline septum divides into halves
  - Tunica albuginea: Fibrous capsule surrounding testicle
    - Mediastinum testis formed by fold of tunica which has variable echogenicity at ultrasound
  - Tunica vaginalis has two layers
    - Visceral layer adherent to tunica albuginea
    - Outer parietal layer normally separated from visceral by small amount of fluid

Scrotal Trauma

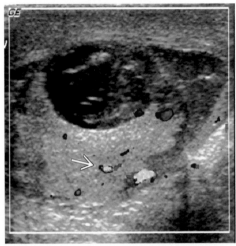

A follow-up ultrasound at two days shows good flow within the testicle. Arrow indicates Doppler flow signal.

- o Epididymis is adjacent to the mediastinum and includes head, body and tail
  - ▪ Head 10-12 mm in size and slightly more echogenic than testis

CT Findings
- Fluid collection in scrotum
- Hematoma in or near scrotum
- Associated pelvic fractures or urethral injury

Ultrasound Findings
- Rupture of testicle
  - o Irregularity of testicular outline (only specific feature of rupture)
  - o Inhomogeneity of testicular texture
  - o Fracture line is seen in only about 17%
  - o Rupture may be missed at ultrasound; hematocele may be only finding
- Hematocele
  - o Occurs in 1/3 of patients with testicular rupture
  - o Looks like hydrocele but with low level echoes
  - o Hydrocele is anechoic excess fluid collection between parietal and visceral layers of tunica vaginalis
- Hematoma of testicle
  - o Inhomogeneously echogenic rounded or oval area within testis
- Tortion
  - o Color Doppler shows asymmetric or absent blood flow
  - o Gray-scale, like in orchitis, may show enlargement and decreased echogenicity or may appear normal acutely
- Dislocation of testis
  - o Abnormal location
  - o Other testicular injuries
- Post traumatic epididymitis
  - o Swollen epididymis with decreased echogenicity
  - o Hyperemia on Doppler is frequent finding

Scrotal Trauma

Imaging Recommendations
- Ultrasound for evaluation of scrotal contents
- Retrograde urethrogram for evaluation of associated urethral injury

Differential Diagnosis
Tumor or Inflammation
- Findings of injury at ultrasound are not specific and must be taken in context of trauma
- 60% of patients with tumor have hydrocele

Pathology
- None relevant to this case

Clinical Issues
Presentation
- Testicular rupture
  - Tenderness, swelling, ecchymosis
- Testicular tortion
  - Tenderness, high-riding position, possibly horizontal lie, swelling
Treatment
- Indications for testicular surgery after trauma
  - Hematocele (may be only finding in rupture)
  - Expanding hematoma
  - Ruptured testis
  - Suspicious clinical findings
- Surgical repair for dislocation and for testicular rupture
- Surgical orchiopexy for torsion
- Ice packs for testicular or scrotal contusion
Prognosis
- Untreated testicular injury can lead to infection, abscess or atrophy
  - Delayed diagnosis results in orchiectomy rate of about 45%
- Prognosis for salvage of testis poor with tortion greater than 6 hours
  - Salvage rate gets progressively worse between 4 and 10 hours
  - About 90% success rate if intervention for rupture occurs before 72 hours, only 45% after 72 hours

Selected References
1. Micallef M et al: Ultrasound features of blunt testicular injury. Injury. 32:23-6, 2001
2. Horstman WG: Scrotal imaging. Urol Clin North Am. 24:653-71, 1997
3. Munter DW et al: Blunt scrotal trauma: emergency department evaluation and management. Am J Emerg Med. 7:227-34, 1989

PocketRadiologist®

ER-Trauma
Top 100 Diagnoses

THORACOLUMBAR SPINE TRAUMA

Thoracolumbar Compression Fract.

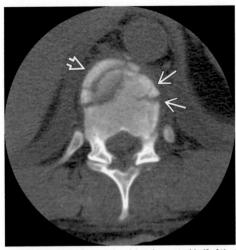

Axial NECT shows comminuted fracture involving the ventral half of the T9 vertebral body. Frank fracture fragments are evident as well as a curvilinear "halo" fragment (open arrow). A thin rim of soft tissue density adjacent to the outer vertebral boarder represents hematoma and edema (arrows).

Key Facts
- Synonym(s): Wedge compression fracture
- Definition: Loss of height in a thoracic or lumbar vertebral body due to a crush fracture of the cortical bone
  - Most commonly a fracture of the anterior-superior end plate
    - Superior lateral end plate compression fracture possible but much less likely
  - Can involve up to 2/3 of the antero-posterior length of the vertebral body (anterior vertebral column)
  - Typically less than 50% loss of total vertebral body height
- Classic imaging appearance: Vertebral body takes on a "wedge-like" appearance on lateral plain film examination
- Other key facts
  - Often related to axial loading while in a flexed position
    - Accounts for 48% of thoracic and lumbar fractures
  - Posterior 1/3 of vertebral body, articulating facets and neural arch NOT fractured
  - Results in pronounced thoracic kyphosis
  - Painful, but mechanically stable fracture

Imaging Findings
General Features
- Best imaging clue: Wedge like appearance of thoracic vertebra on lateral projection
- Other generic features: Ratio of anterior to posterior vertebral body height when measured from the lateral projection is considered normal if 80% or greater in females and 85% or greater in males
- Superior end plate anteriorly depressed
  - Subtle sclerotic impaction line may be evident parallel to the compressed section

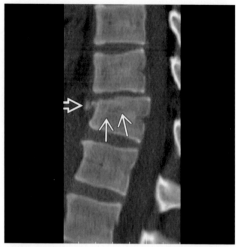

Sagittal CT reformation shows asymmetrical loss of height in the anterior T9 vertebral body with mild depression of the superior end plate, fragment "beak" (open arrow) and subtle hyperdense line paralleling the depressed segment (arrows). Mild pronouncement in the thoracic kyphosis is noted.

CT Findings

- Axial CT
  - "Halo" of fragmented bone may surround the anterior curvature of the fractured vertebra
  - Posterior cortex between the pedicles and neural arch INTACT
  - Soft tissue hematoma and edema associated with the endplate involved
- Sagittal CT reformations
  - Loss of anterior vertebral body height
  - Fragment "beak" may be present
  - Sclerotic impaction line parallels depressed superior end plate segment

MR Findings

- T1WI
  - Asymmetric low signal in the marrow space adjacent to the depressed segment
- T2WI
  - Hyperintense signal in the marrow space paralleling the depressed superior end plate segment

Imaging Recommendations

- A lateral plain film will often recognize the characteristic appearance
- Further imaging with CT may be necessary to separate a simple anterior compression from a burst fracture
- MRI may help define marrow space edema suggesting subacute from chronic time course, but edema and hemorrhage are slow to resolve, resulting in vague results
  - DWI to differentiate metastatic vs. osteoporotic disease CONTROVERSIAL

- o Prior films for comparison most accurate when trying to differentiate acute from chronic
- o Nuclear medicine bone scan may be helpful in detecting multiple levels

Differential Diagnosis
Thoracic Burst Fracture
- May have similar overall gross appearance, but fracture extends to the posterior vertebral cortex and retropulsed fragments are seen in the vertebral canal

Limbus Vertebra
- An accessory ossification center at the anterior superior margin of the vertebra results in a separate, well-defined wedge of cortical bone

Scheuermann's Kyphosis (Congenital Round Back)
- Represents an asymmetry in growth between the anterior and posterior vertebral body in young males
- Typically apex at T7-T9

Pathology
General
- General Path Comments
  - o Loss of bony integrity of the vertebral body by infiltrating or destructive lesions (lymphoma, metastases) or loss of mineral matrix (osteoporosis) increases the likelihood of failure of the vertebra in compression
- Etiology-Pathogenesis
  - o Increased compressive stress on the ventral vertebral body anterior to the nucleus pulposus overcomes the structural integrity of the ventral cortical bone causing it to fail

Clinical Issues
Presentation
- Severe back pain following hyperflexion or hyperflexed axial loading
- May result in pronounced kyphosis specially if multiple and chronic intermittent

Treatment
- Typically symptomatic treatment only
- Consider percutaneous vertebroplasty in severe painful osteoporosis

Selected References
1. Old JL, et al: Vertebral compression fractures in the elderly. Am Fam Physician 69(1):111-6, 2004
2. Jung HS, et al: Discrimination of metastatic from acute osteoporotic compression spinal fractures with MR imaging. Radiographics 23(1):179-87, 2003
3. Zhou XJ, et al: Characterization of benign and metastatic vertebral compression fractures with quantitative diffusion MR imaging. AJNR Am J Neuroradiol 23(1):165-70, 2002

Thoracolumbar Burst Fracture

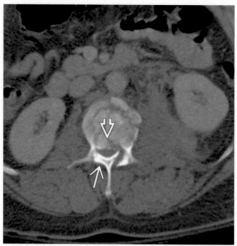

Axial CT shows a comminuted fracture of the ventral, lateral and dorsal cortex of the L2 vertebral body. The neural arch is also fractured at the bilateral lamina. The central canal is compressed by dorsally displaced vertebral body fragments (open arrow) and an anteriorly displaced neural arch fragment (arrow).

Key Facts
- Synonym(s): Unstable compression fracture
- Definition: Comminuted fracture of the thoracic vertebral body (VB) that extends through both the superior and inferior endplates
  - Fracture extends through the ventral and posterior cortex
    - Ventral ½ of VB = anterior column (AC)
    - Posterior ½ of VB to pedicle = middle column (MC)
    - May also involve posterior column (neural arch), but not necessary for diagnosis
  - KEY: Involvement of MC differentiates this fracture from stable anterior wedge compression fracture
- Classic imaging appearance: Loss of vertebral height and widening of both the inter pedicle distance and antero-posterior length
- UNSTABLE fracture
  - Loss of weight bearing strength of VB due to destruction of structural integrity of the bony cortex
  - Anterior and posterior longitudinal ligaments (ALL/PLL) injured by definition since they are in close approximation the VB
    - Contributes to instability
- Displaced fragments may impinge on local structures
  - Spinal canal, aorta, IVC

Imaging Findings
General Features
- Best imaging clue: Loss of VB height, widened interpedicle distance
  - Fragment may be displaced into spinal canal on lateral view
CT Findings
- Axial images with sagittal reformations a MUST, coronal optional

Thoracolumbar Burst Fracture

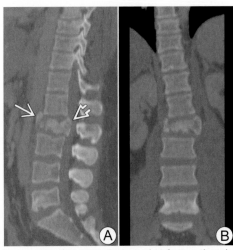

Sagittal and coronal CT reformations show complete fracture through the superior and inferior endplate (A, arrow) and "buckled" dorsally displaced fragment (A, open arrow). Coronal reformation (B) shows fragmentation, loss of height and apex leftward angulation.

- Axial: comminuted fracture with fragments pushed radially away from the center of the VB
  - May create a "halo" of fragments
  - Can lead to confusion with stable anterior wedge compression
- Sagittal: AP widening of the VB with loss of height
  - Anterior and posterior spinal line deviations
  - Fragment may be displaced into spinal canal
  - Adjacent hematoma may also invade spinal canal
- Coronal: Lateral displacement of fragments
  - Increased inter-pedicle distance

MR Findings
- T1WI findings relate to destruction of VB
  - Anatomic findings similar to CT
  - Marrow space heterogeneous or uniform decreased signal
    - Marrow space edema and hemorrhage
- T2WI reflect edema and hemorrhage in the cord, VB marrow space, peri-vertebral space and epidural space of spinal canal
  - Increased signal in VB marrow space, peri-vertebral soft tissues and epidural space of spinal canal
- Gradient echo susceptibility WI increases sensitivity for detecting hemorrhagic material in all vertebral spaces and in the cord

Imaging Recommendations
- Initial workup should be CT including sagittal reformations
- Consider MRI for canal evaluation
  - Essential if neurological symptoms

Differential Diagnosis

Stable Compression Fracture (Anterior Wedge Compression)
- Loss of height in anterior column only

Thoracolumbar Burst Fracture

- Does NOT extend to middle column
- Usually only fracture of the superior endplate

Pathology
General
- Usually the result of direct axial loading to normal VB
  - Force dropped on head
  - Jump from height, landing on feet
  - Hard fall onto buttocks in sitting position
- In compromised VB, may occur spontaneously or with little force
  - Destructive expansile or infiltrative metastatic disease
  - NOT likely in simple osteoporosis which more likely leads to simple anterior wedge or central endplate depression

Clinical Issues
Presentation
- 60% occur between T12-L2; 90% occur between T11-L4
  - Thoracolumbar junction vulnerable due to transition from rib-bearing, smaller vertebra structure to non-rib bearing, larger
- 65% associated with neurological deficit
  - Paralysis, sensory deficit distal to cord injury
Treatment
- Aimed at restoring weight bearing mechanical stability and resolving cord compression by fragments or hematoma
  - Surgical stabilization with fixation or fusion
  - Surgical decompression of spinal canal
  - Non-surgical treatment (bedrest, brace) in selected MILD cases
Prognosis
- If cord injury is present, depends on degree of injury
  - Cord transection - poor neurological prognosis
  - Cord contusion – variable neurological prognosis

Selected References
1. Yue JJ, et al: The treatment of unstable thoracic spine fractures with transpedicular screw instrumentation: A 3-year consecutive series. Spine. 27(24):2782-7, 2002
2. Kim NH, et al: Neurologic injury and recovery in patients with burst fracture of the thoracolumbar spine. Spine. 1;24(3):290-3, 1999
3. Petersilge CA, et al: Thoracolumbar burst fractures: Evaluation with MR imaging. Radiology. 194(1):49-54, 1995

Thoracic Facet Dislocation

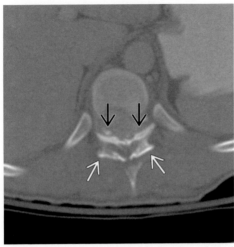

Axial NECT shows superior facet (white arrows) dorsal to inferior facets (black arrows). The facet joints are widened. Note that the flat articulating surface of the facets are on the outside, facing away from the joint and the rounded surfaces face inward giving a bilateral "naked facet" appearance.

Key Facts
- Synonyms: Jumped facet, locked facet, perched facet
- Definition: Derangement of the facet joint configuration so that positioning of the superior and inferior facets is reversed
- Classic imaging appearance: Superior and inferior facet positions, reversed, asymmetrically widened posterior disk space and anterolisthesis of the vertebral body associated with the displaced inferior facet
  - Sometimes accompanied by widened inter-spinous process and inter-laminar distance, mildly pronounced kyphosis, vertebral body rotation and anterolisthesis of the vertebral body associated with the displaced inferior facet
  - Other key facts
    - Pure forms of both the uni- and bilateral facet dislocation without vertebral body fracture are uncommon in the thoracic spine
    - Unilateral facet dislocation if mechanism is hyperflexion-rotation
    - Both facets may be displaced forced hyperflexion without rotation
    - The smaller superior facet may fracture during displacement
    - Fragment may impinge on spinal nerve

Imaging Findings
General Features
- Best imaging clue: Visualization of reversed superior and inferior facets
  - Other generic features: Asymmetrically widened posterior disk space, widened inter-spinous process distance, mildly pronounced kyphosis, vertebral body rotation and anterolisthesis of the

Thoracic Facet Dislocation

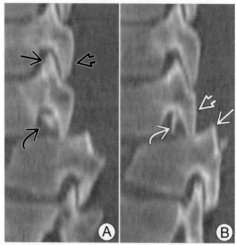

Sagittal CT shows normal facet joint with superior facet (A, black arrow) antero-inferior to inferior facet (A, open black arrow). Dislocation shows reversal with superior facet (B, white arrow) now postero-inferior to inferior facet (B, open white arrow). There is a fracture fragment in the neural foramen (curved black arrows).

CT Findings
- NECT On axial images, joint appears widened
- Normally, flat surface of facets articulate inward with rounded surface facing away from joint
- Jumped facet shows reversal of this architecture, with the rounded part of on the inside and the flat surface on the outside = "naked facet" appearance
- Sagittal reformations show inferior facet of the more cephalad vertebra "jumped" over the superior facet of the lower vertebra
- May result in anterolisthesis of the upper on lower vertebra
- Coronal and axial views may show slight rotation of the upper vertebral body in a unilateral jumped facet

MR Findings
- T1WI Anatomic changes as above
- Low signal marrow space edema
- T2WI Hyperintensity in soft tissues surrounding the jumped facet may indicate strain of the capsular ligaments, ligamenta flava or interspinous ligaments
- T2WI and gradient echo susceptibility imaging are critical to evaluation of the spinal canal and cord

Imaging Recommendations
- CT with reformation is key to making the diagnosis
- MRI is critical to evaluate canal, cord and ligaments

Differential Diagnosis

Thoracic Fracture Dislocation
- Fracture dislocation much more common than dislocation without fracture
- Axial compression or moment of inertial resulting from distracting forces usually result in vertebral body compression

Thoracic Facet Dislocation

Pathology
General
- Ligaments undergo tensile stress when facet is dislocated
  - Capsular ligaments torn
  - Posterior longitudinal ligament, ligamentum flavum, interspinous and supraspinous ligaments may also be torn
- Etiology-Pathogenesis
  - Hyperflexion without axial loading
  - The fulcrum of force is placed anterior to the vertebral body resulting in forced distraction of the posterior elements
    - Forced distraction with failure of the posterior ligamentous complex (PLC = capsular ligaments, ligamentum flavum, interspinous ligament and supraspinous ligament)

Clinical Issues
Presentation
- Focal back pain with limited range of extensor motion (if locked and not fractured)
- May present with neurological sequelae (paralysis, sensory deficit) in 60-70% of cases
Treatment
- Traction to reduce dislocated facets
- Surgical fusion may be necessary to stabilize compromised ligaments
Prognosis
- Good if no associated neurological injury and mechanically stable

Selected References
1. Lucas MJ, et al: Unilateral thoracic facet dislocation. Clin Orthop. (335):162-5, 1997
2. Sharafuddin MJ, et al: Locked facets in the thoracic spine: report of three cases and a review. J Spinal Disord. 3(3):255-8, 1990
3. Levine AM, et al: Bilateral facet dislocations in the thoracolumbar spine. Spine. 13(6):630-40, 1988

Thoracic Distraction (Chance) Fx

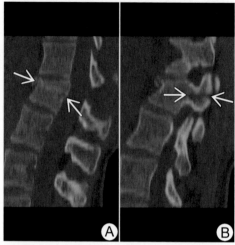

Thoracic flexion distraction fracture type I (Chance fracture). Arrows show fracture line through the pedicle and facet complex (B), continuing through the entire vertebral body in this case (A). Note anterior compression type appearance of the ventral vertebral body.

Key Facts
- Synonyms: Seatbelt fracture, hyperflexion-distraction fracture
- Definition: Horizontally oriented fracture through the neural arch with partial or complete extension to involve the vertebral body
  - Neural arch = pedicle, facets, laminae and spinous process
- Classic imaging appearance "wedged" or "compressed" vertebral body with distracted or split neural arch elements
- Occur principally at thoraco-lumbar junction (T11-L2), but may be lower (L2-L4) in children
- More prevalent in children than adults
  - Lower center of gravity
  - 3-point restraint worn as 2-point OR unrestrained child flies forward, striking abdomen on back of front seat in MVC
    - 2-point (lap) belt slides over superior iliac crest and a narrow line of force is applied across the abdomen
    - Results in hyper flexion with shearing force simultaneously driven into abdomen
- High degree of associated abdominal organ injury - up to 50% in children

Imaging Findings
General Features
- Best imaging clue: Anterior angulation or compression fracture appearance
- In general, alignment is preserved in this type of injury
- Splayed neural arch elements may not be obvious on plain film
Plain Film Features
- AP: Missing spinous process – "empty" vertebra
- Lateral: Anterior angulation and loss of vertebral body height
  - Splayed posterior elements with or without fracture line evident

Thoracic Distraction (Chance) Fx

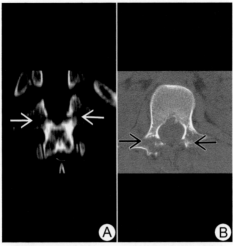

Fracture through the neural arch in coronal and axial projection. (A) shows a fracture line (between arrows) dividing the pedicle at its junction with the transverse process. (B) shows the same fracture line (between arrows) in the axial plane. Fracture line is parallel to image plane in axial view.

CT Findings
- Horizontal fracture through spinous process
- Fracture extends through articulations, transverse processes and pedicles
- Horizontal fracture continues into vertebral body
- Blurred epidural fat plane in the spinal canal or para-vertebral soft tissues implies traction injury to soft tissue

MR Findings
- T1WI Iso to slightly hyperintense hematoma may be seen
  - Alignment is usually maintained as fracture passes through vertebra and leaves ligaments intact
- T2WI with fat suppression shows hyperintensity in ligamentum flavum
  - Supra and interspinous ligaments, anterior and posterior longitudinal ligaments, capsular ligaments and annulus fibrosis may be normal or slightly hyperintense.
  - Cord normal – neurological injury not common (~ 20%)

Imaging Recommendations
- CT with coronal, sagittal and if possible 3-D reformations VERY helpful

Differential Diagnosis

Simple (Anterior Wedge) Compression Fracture
- Anterior vertebral body fractured, but not neural arch

Burst fracture
- Whole vertebral body fractured, but not neural arch

Jumped Facet
- Anterior angulation
- Facet misplaced and may be fractured, but lamina, pedicle and transverse and spinous processes are not

Thoracic Distraction (Chance) Fx

Fracture-Dislocation
- Vertebral body fractured and facets displaced, but neural arch intact

Pathology
General
- Forced flexion with fulcrum anterior to the vertebra (i.e., seat belt) which imparts a distracting force to the vertebra and neural arch
  - Spinous process fails in tension, splitting horizontally
  - Distracting force transferred to lamina which split horizontally
  - Force continues through articulating facets and transverse processes
  - Pedicles split, delivering distracting force closer to the fulcrum
  - Fulcrum itself (vertebra) splits to varying degrees, part to complete

Types
- Chance (type I) Fracture through spinous process, laminae, articulating facet complex, transverse processes, pedicles and variable vertebral body
- Smith (type II) Same as type I, but does not split spinous process, but instead tears interspinous and suprasinous ligaments

Clinical Issues
Presentation
- ALL FLEXION-DISTRACTION TYPE FRACTURES ARE CONSIDERED UNSTABLE
- Neurological injury in only 20% of flexion-distraction cases

Selected References
1. Renne W et al: Flexion distraction fractures of the thoracolumbar spine. J Bone Joint Surg Am. 55:386, 1973
2. Rogers LF: The roentgenographic appearance of transverse or Chance fractures of the spine: The seat belt fracture. AJR. 111:844, 1971
3. Smith WS et al: Patterns and mechanisms of Lumbar injuries associated with lap seat belts. J Bone Joint Surg AM. 51:239, 1969

Thoracic Fracture Dislocation

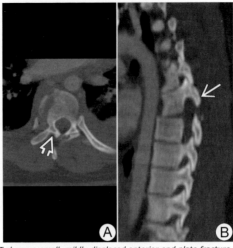

(A) Axial CT shows a small, mildly displaced anterior end plate fracture and "naked" right facet (arrow). (B) A perched facet (arrow) with anterior angulation and accentuated kyphosis is best appreciated on sagittal CT reformation. Coronal reformations may help define any lateral translation.

Key Facts
- Synonym: Translation injury
- Definition: Destruction of the structural integrity of the vertebral body, supporting ligaments and articulating joints following a combination of flexion, axial loading and rotational forces
- Classic imaging appearance
  - Anterior displacement of the vertebral body above the injury
  - Some degree of compression may be present in the superior endplate of the vertebra below the injury
  - A triangular fragment is commonly sheared from the anterior superior margin of the lower vertebral body
  - The posterior ligament complex (PLC - interspinous, supraspinous and capsular ligaments and ligamentum flavum) is variably disrupted and the superior facet of the lower vertebra is dislocated or sheared off
  - Perched or locked facets are common
  - Less commonly, lateral or posterior translation may be apparent
- Other key facts
  - All three columns of the spine and the supporting ligaments are involved
    - Inherently UNSTABLE injury

Imaging Findings
General Features
- Best imaging clue: Mal-alignment of the spine with anterolisthesis of the vertebra above the injury
- Spinal canal compromise is evident; normal articulation of facet joints cannot be seen
- Neural arch may be obviously fractured

Thoracic Fracture Dislocation

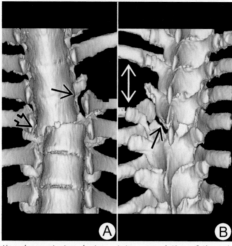

3D reformation demonstrates dextro-rotatory angulation of thoracic spine with separation of transverse process from pedicle (A, arrow) and small anterior fracture fragment (A, open arrow). Perched left facet joint (B, arrow) and widened intercostal space (B, double arrow) is evident posteriorly.

<u>CT Findings</u>
- Axial images demonstrate findings similar to compression type fractures of the vertebral body (Comminution, "Halo" fragments)
- Normal "sandwich" appearance of the thoracic facet joint not seen
- May see one facet, then another as you scroll down images ("naked" facet) or reversal of the articulating facet surfaces (jumped or locked facet)
- May not visualize facet at all if sheared off
  - Look for free fragments
- Sagittal reformations show mal-alignment with anterolisthesis of the upper on lower vertebral bodies
- Sagittal imaging may show widened interspinous or interlaminar spaces
- Soft tissue hematoma may be present if injury to supra or interspinous ligament, ligamentum flavum or capsular ligaments

<u>MR Findings</u>
- Anatomic relations apparent on T1 and T2WI as described in CT section
- Marrow space signal abnormality at site of fracture reflects marrow edema with diminished T1 and increased T2 signal in close approximation to the fracture of vertebral body and/or facet
- Edema and hemorrhage in ligament injury, particularly interspinous ligament evident as increased T2WI signal
  - Fat suppressed imaging is vital to recognition of this signal abnormality as fat interspersed with ligament fibers will give increased signal that will obscure abnormal signal
  - Occasionally, complete tear of ligament will demonstrate free edge of low signal ligament fibers against hemorrhage/edema hyperintensity

Thoracic Fracture Dislocation

- Cord injury should be evaluated with T2WI, gradient echo susceptibility (GRE), and/or, if available diffusion weighted imaging (DWI)
  - Hyperintense T2WI cord edema and hemorrhage
  - Hemorrhage revealed as iso to hypointense GRE signal
  - Restricted diffusion (hyperintense DWI) suggests cord cell injury – DWI findings currently investigative and controversial

Imaging Recommendations
- Plain films are often limited, especially in the upper thoracic spine
  - Good for a first survey, but often need additional detail
- NECT with Sagittal and coronal reformations are essential
- MRI for assessment of cord injury and ligamentous injury

Differential Diagnosis
Flexion-Distraction (Chance or Smith) Injury
- Horizontal split in neural arch
- Facets NOT dislocated or jumped, but split
- Little of no vertebral compression

Facet Dislocation (Locked or Perched Facet)
- Injury to vertebral body is minimal
- Facet fracture may be present, but mainly facet is dislocated or jumped
- PLC may be injured, but ALL and PLL may be intact
- Better chance of maintaining overall structural integrity

Pathology
- None relevant to this case

Clinical Issues
Presentation
- Flexion, axial loading and rotation mechanism
- Severe back pain, deformation
- Most common at T4-5 or T5-6 levels
- If injury in T5-T8 segment, almost always neurological symptoms
  - Most commonly complete motor and sensory deficit, but may be as subtle as central cord syndrome

Treatment
- Surgical reduction of fracture and decompression of spinal canal
- Pedicle screw fixation and bone graft fusion to stabilize spine

Prognosis
- Up to 75% may present with neurological deficit
  - Up to 50% of these will be complete with poor outcome
- If no initial neurological deficit, up to 90% may return to full function

Selected References
1. el-Khoury GY et al: Trauma to the upper thoracic spine: anatomy, biomechanics, and unique imaging features. AJR Am J Roentgenol. 160(1):95-102, 1993
2. Manaster BJ et al: CT patterns of facet fracture dislocations in the thoracolumbar region. AJR Am J Roentgenol. 148(2): 335-40, 1987
3. Denis F: The three-column spine and its significance in the classification of acute thoracolumbar spinal injuries. Spine 8:817, 1983

PocketRadiologist®

ER-Trauma
Top 100 Diagnoses

UPPER EXTREMITY INJURY

Clavicle Fracture

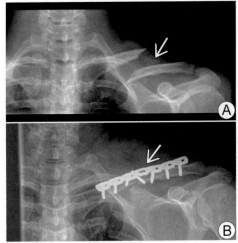

Clavicle fracture. (A) Clavicle film demonstrates classic fracture of the midshaft of clavicle with inferior and medial displacement of distal fracture fragment (arrow). (B) Same patient, status post open reduction and internal fixation of the fracture with near anatomic alignment (arrow).

Key Facts
- Synonym: Disrupted collarbone
- Definition: Break of the clavicle bone
- Classic imaging appearance: Lucency through the clavicle bone
- Other key facts
  - Most commonly results from direct fall on the shoulder
  - Most frequent fracture site in children
  - Can occur at birth during passage through the birth canal
  - Middle third of the clavicle involved in approximately 80% of cases

Imaging Findings
General Features
- Best imaging clue: Transverse and complete fracture of the middle third
- Distal fragment of clavicle displaces inferiorly and medially
- Other generic features: Sigmoid shaped clavicle bone with two articulations at both proximal and distal ends
- Anatomy
  - Muscle attachments to almost the entire inferior and superior surfaces of clavicle
    - Short segment in the midportion free of attachment
  - Strong ligamentous support distally and proximally
Radiography Findings
- AP clavicle: Visible transverse and complete break in the cortex with inferior and medial displacement of the distal fracture fragment
  - In childhood often a greenstick or bowing type fracture
- Stress view of the clavicle with weights: Evaluation of the integrity of the distal ligaments most importantly coracoclavicular ligament
CT Findings
- Evaluation of displaced interligamentous fractures

Clavicle Fracture

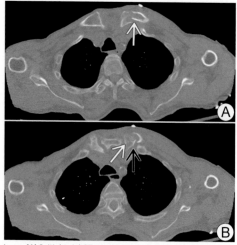

Clavicle fracture. (A) Initial axial CT scan through the chest demonstrates comminuted fracture of the proximal clavicle (arrow). (B) Same patient, further distal axial images again show the comminuted fracture (black arrow). Note that the sternoclavicular joint is preserved (white arrow).

- Evaluation of questionable fracture of medial third

MR Findings
- T1WI: Linear dark signal fracture line
  - T1WI fat-sat: Evaluation of osteolysis
- T2WI: Linear high signal fracture line
- Ligamentous injuries

Imaging Recommendations
- Initial detection of clavicle fracture by radiography
- CT indicated in cases of intraarticular distal third fractures
- MRI is indicated for evaluation of soft tissue injuries

Differential Diagnosis
Medial Clavicular Epiphysis
- Medial epiphyseal margin may mimic avulsion fracture
- Last epiphysis to ossify and fuse, may occur as late as 25 years of age
- Differentiated from clavicle fracture by location and margins

Pathology
- None relevant to this case

Clinical Issues
Presentation
- Pain and swelling overlying clavicle

Treatment
- Fracture of the mid clavicle: Sling or figure-of-eight bandage
- Fracture of the proximal third: Sling
- Fracture of the distal third
  - Stable: Sling
  - Unstable: Open reduction and internal fixation

Clavicle Fracture

<u>Prognosis</u>
- Most clavicular fractures heal without complications
- Rarely complications (1-4% of cases)
  - Nonunion
  - Underlying subclavian artery, vein or brachial plexus injury
  - Pneumothorax
  - Post-traumatic osteolysis

Selected References
1. Stanley D et al: The mechanism of clavicular fracture. A clinical and biomechanical analysis. J. Bone Joint Surg. 70:461, 1988
2. Heppenstall RB: Fractures and dislocations of the distal clavicle. Orthop. Clin. North Am. 6:477, 1975
3. Sankarankutty M et al: Fractures of the clavicle. Injury. 7:101, 1975

Acromioclavicular Separation

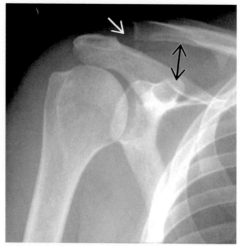

Acromioclavicular separation. AP radiograph of the right shoulder demonstrates widening (arrow) of the acromioclavicular joint as well as increased coracoclavicular distance (double arrow) consistent with type III injury.

Key Facts
- Synonym: Acromioclavicular dislocation, shoulder separation
- Definition: Disruption of the acromioclavicular (A-C) ligaments with or without injury to the coracoclavicular (C-C) ligaments
- Classic imaging appearance: Widening of the acromioclavicular joint space with or without widening of the coracoclavicular distance
- Associated with fractures of
  - Coracoid process
  - Distal end of the clavicle

Imaging Findings
General Features
- Best imaging clue: Widening of the acromioclavicular joint
  - Comparison with the contra-lateral side should be made before establishing the diagnosis
- Classification
  - Type I: Mild, bruised ligaments, no actual separation of the AC joint
  - Type II: Moderate, partial tear in the acromioclavicular ligaments, slight separation of the A-C joint
  - Type III: Severe, complete tear of the acromio- as well as the coracoclavicular ligaments, complete separation of the AC joint
  - Type IV: Type III injury and associated posterior dislocation of the distal end of the clavicle
- Anatomy: The joint is supported by
  - Thin fibrous capsule
  - Discrete acromioclavicular ligaments (anteriorly, posteriorly, superiorly, and inferiorly)
  - Coracoclavicular ligaments

Acromioclavicular Separation

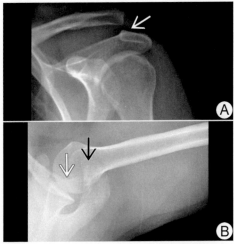

Acromioclavicular separation. (A) AP view of the left shoulder shows widening of the A-C joint (arrow) with increased C-C distance. (B) Type IV injury: Axillary view of the left shoulder in the same patient demonstrates posterior dislocation of the distal clavicle (white arrow). Acromion is in its normal position (black arrow).

Radiography Findings
- AP shoulder: Difference between the acromioclavicular joint from side to side no more than 2 mm with or without coracoclavicular widening
- Weight bearing AP of both shoulders: Evaluation of instability

CT Findings
- Evaluation of associated fractures
- Evaluation of the degree of injury

MR Findings
- T1WI: Low signal edema
- T2WI: High signal edema
- Evaluation of associated ligamentous and muscle injuries

Imaging Recommendations
- Best seen on modified AP view with the beam angled 10-15 degrees cephalad
- Posterior dislocation of distal clavicle (type IV separation) best appreciated on axillary views
- Contralateral joint should always be imaged for comparison, because of wide variations in normal anatomy
- Preferably second similar radiograph should be obtained with arm hanging loosely with 10 to 15 pound weights in each hand for evaluation of instability

Differential Diagnosis

Pseudodislocation of the Acromio-Clavicular Joint
- Fracture-separation of the distal margin of the clavicle, giving the clinical and radiological appearance of a complete acromioclavicular dislocation

Panclavicular Dislocations
- Simultaneous dislocation of the acromioclavicular and sternoclavicular joints

Acromioclavicular Separation

<u>Os Acromiale</u>
- Normal variant may mimic widening of the acromioclavicular joint

Pathology
<u>General</u>
- Etiology-Pathogenesis
  - Downward blow to the clavicle (sports related)
  - Applying traction to the arm
  - Falling on the hand or elbow with the arm flexed at a 90 degree angulation

Clinical Issues
<u>Presentation</u>
- Acromioclavicular pain with joint deformity in the form of a prominent "lump" that can be seen and felt
- Limited movement of the shoulder
- Swelling and bruising

<u>Treatment</u>
- Type I: Sling and adhesive strapping
- Type II: Same as above may or may not require arthroplasty
- Type III: Internal fixation; fixation screw being passed from the clavicle downwards into the coracoid process
- Type IV: Open reduction and internal fixation

<u>Prognosis</u>
- Type I: Excellent
- Type II: 90% recover, 10% require surgery
- Type III: 80% good, 20% reoperation
- Type IV: Similar to type III

Selected References
1.   Clarke HD et al: Acromioclavicular joint injuries. Orthop. Clin. North Am. 31:177, 2000
2.   Phillips AM et al: Acromioclavicular dislocation. Conservative or surgical therapy. Clin. Orthop. 353:10, 1998
3.   Keats TE et al: The acromioclavicular joint: Normal variation and the diagnosis of dislocation. Skeletal Radiol. 17:159, 1988

Anterior Shoulder Dislocation

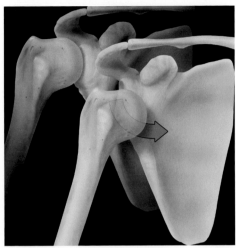

Drawing illustrates position of humeral head with anterior shoulder dislocation.

Key Facts
- Synonyms: Anterior glenohumeral dislocation
- Definition: Dislocation of the humeral head relative to the glenoid fossa, resulting in complete loss of continuity of joint surfaces
- Humeral head lies medial, and inferior to glenoid on AP view, and anterior to glenoid on lateral view
- Most common type of shoulder dislocation
- May be associated with a compression fracture of the humeral head (i.e., Hill-Sachs lesion), and/or the glenoid labrum (i.e., Bankart lesion)

Imaging Findings
General Features
- Best imaging clue: Humeral head does not articulate properly with the glenoid fossa
- Other generic features: Humeral head typically lies inferior and medially

CT Findings
- Essentially the same as for plain film
- Hill-Sachs and Bankart lesions may be better shown by CT

MR Findings
- T2WI may show synovial fluid (high signal) dissecting underneath the glenoid labrum if a Bankart lesion is present, or into the supraspinatus tendon, indicating the presence of a rotator cuff tear

Other Modality Findings
- Labral and rotator cuff tears may be visible on shoulder arthrogram

Imaging Recommendations
- Check pre an post reduction films
- Obtain Stryker notch view to detect a Hill-Sachs lesion
- Obtain Westpoint axillary view to detect a Bankart fracture
- CT or MR may detect Hill-Sachs or Bankart lesions not seen on plane films, and should be obtain if high suspicion exists

Anterior Shoulder Dislocation

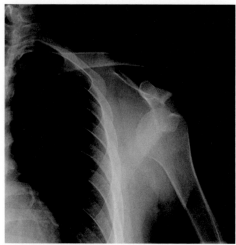

This AP film of the left shoulder shows the typical appearance of an anterior glenohumeral dislocation. The humeral head lies inferior and medial to the glenoid. The lateral view would confirm the anterior position of the humeral head.

Differential Diagnosis
Anterior Shoulder Subluxation
- Chronic condition
- Patient may have history of recurrent shoulder dislocations
- Humeral head remains partially articulated with the glenoid fossa

Pathology
General
- Etiology-Pathogenesis
  - Fall on an abducted, externally rotated arm, driving humeral head anteriorly
- Epidemiology
  - Most commonly dislocated joint in the body
  - Shoulder dislocations account for 85% of all dislocations in the body
  - 95% of all shoulder dislocations are anterior
Gross Pathologic, Surgical Features
- Arthoscopy may show torn labrum, loose bodies, and/or rotator cuff tear

Clinical Issues
Presentation
- History of trauma with abduction and external rotation of upper extremity
- Patient holds affected arm close to his body in external rotation
- Anterior fullness of the shoulder to palpation
- Hill-Sachs lesion present in 60% of patients with primary dislocation
- Rotator cuff tears present in 50% of patients < 40 y and 80% in those > 60 y
- Occasionally nerve damage (axillary > posterior cord > musculocutaneous) resulting from traction

Anterior Shoulder Dislocation

Treatment
- Reduction by various techniques (e.g., external rotation, Stimson's technique)
- Sling
- Physical therapy and early mobilization to prevent frozen shoulder
- Surgery if necessary to correct recurrent shoulder instability

Prognosis
- Depends on presence of associated injuries
- Bankart lesion (avulsion of the anteroinferior glenoid labrum at its attachment to the inferior glenohumeral ligament) present in 90% of patients with primary dislocation, and often requires surgical repair to prevent recurrent instability
- Recurrent dislocations more common in patients who sustain initial injury at younger ages 80-90% (< 2 y), 10-15% (> 40 y)
- 20% of patients have intraarticular loose bodies, significant cartilaginous injury leading to persistent pain, mechanical symptoms or arthropathy at 10 years
- Nerve injury may take months to resolve

Selected References
1. Wischer TK et al: Perthes lesion (a variant of the Bankart lesion): MR imaging and MR arthrographic findings with surgical correlation. AJR. 178(1):233-7, 2002
2. Tuckman GA et al: Axillary nerve injury after anterior glenohumeral dislocation: MR findings in three patients. AJR. 167(3):695-7, 1996
3. Richards RD et al: Hill-Sachs lesion and normal humeral groove: MR imaging features allowing their differentiation. Radiology. 190(3):665-8, 1994

Posterior Shoulder Dislocation

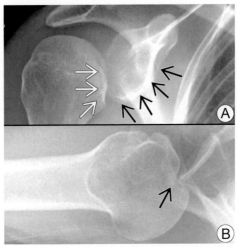

Posterior shoulder dislocation. (A) AP view of the shoulder demonstrates a widened joint space with rim and empty glenoid signs (black arrows); also trough defect is demonstrated (white arrows). (B) Axillary view of the shoulder shows posterior fracture-dislocation of the humeral head (arrow).

Key Facts
- Synonym: Posterior glenohumeral joint disruption
- Definition: Posterior and superior displacement of the humeral head
- Classic imaging appearance
  - Humeral head looks rounded on AP view and posterior to the glenoid fossa on axillary view
  - Persistent internal rotation of the humeral head
- Associated with
  - Detachment of posterior glenoid labrum (reverse Bankhart)
  - Defect of the anteromedial aspect of the humeral head (reverse Hill-Sachs)
  - Fractures of the humeral tuberosities, shaft and/or humeral neck
- Shoulder instability: Frequent dislocations

Imaging Findings
General Features
- Other generic features
  - Light bulb sign: Humeral head looks rounded, like a light bulb
  - Empty glenoid sign: Increased distance between the articular surface of the humeral head and the anterior lip of the glenoid
    - Also called the rim sign: Normal range: 0-6 mm
  - Through defect: Curved dense line, indicating impaction fracture of the antero-medial surface of the humeral head
- Anatomy: Internal rotators overpower the external rotators
  - Internal rotators (subscapularis, latissimus dorsi, pectoralis major)
  - External rotators (teres minor and infraspinatus)
Radiography Findings
- AP view of the shoulder
  - Through defect of the anteromedial humeral head
  - Superior or posterior dislocation

Posterior Shoulder Dislocation

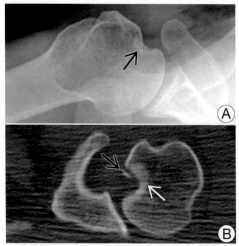

Posterior shoulder dislocation. (A) Axillary radiograph through the shoulder, post reduction, shows the reverse Hill-Sachs defect (arrow). (B) Axial CT image through the shoulder in a different patient obtained post reduction shows reverse Hill-Sachs (white arrow) with a loose fracture fragment (black arrow).

- Axillary view of the shoulder
  - Humeral head lying posterior to the glenoid
  - Posterior glenoid rim fractures

CT Findings
- Reverse Hill-Sachs defect
- Reverse bony Bankhart
- Relation of the articular surfaces, intra-articular fragments

MR Findings
- T1WI
  - Reverse Hill-Sachs defect with dark rim
- T2WI
  - Reverse Bankhart defect: Areas of high signal intensity within glenoid labrum
  - Ligament and muscle injuries: High signal within the injured tissues
- MR arthrography
  - Study of choice for
    - Labral and ligamentous pathology
    - Rotator cuff and cartilage tears

Imaging Recommendations
- Routine radiographs: Anteroposterior (AP) and axillary views
  - Scapular Y view if axillary view can not be obtained
- MDCT
  - 2.5 mm axial
    - Soft tissue and bone algorithm
  - Sagittal and coronal reformations
- MRI
  - Conventional shoulder MR
  - MR arthrogram

Posterior Shoulder Dislocation

Differential Diagnosis
Anterior Shoulder Dislocation
- Humeral head anterior and inferior in relation to the glenoid

Frozen Shoulder
- Limited range of motion in the shoulder with unknown cause
- Develops slowly as oppose to sudden dislocation

Pathology
General
- Etiology-Pathogenesis
  - Axial load to the adducted and internally rotated arm (fall on an outstretched arm or a blow to the front of the shoulder)
  - Electrocution or seizures
- Epidemiology
  - Posterior dislocations: 2-10% of all shoulder dislocations

Clinical Issues
Presentation
- Pain, swelling
- Arm internally rotated and adducted (stiff shoulder)
- A posterior prominence is usually palpable
- The anterior shoulder is flattened

Natural History
- Chronic, repetitive posterior shoulder dislocations
- Degenerative disease of the shoulder

Treatment
- Closed reduction
- Operative repair if closed reduction is unsuccessful

Prognosis
- Often excellent if detected early
- The treated dislocated shoulder is, still very susceptible to reinjury and repeated dislocations, if detected late

Selected References
1. Perron AD et al: Posterior shoulder dislocation: Avoiding a missed diagnosis. Am J Emerg Med. 18:189-91, 2000
2. Elberger ST et al: Bilateral posterior shoulder dislocations. Am J Emerg Med. 13:331-2, 1995
3. Wolfgang GL et al: Roentgenographic recognition of fracture dislocation of shoulder. Orthop. Rev. 11:149, 1982

Proximal Humeral Fracture

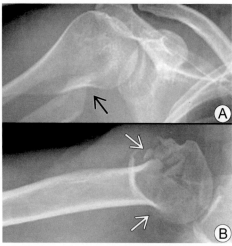

Proximal humeral fracture. (A) Initial AP radiograph of the humerus demonstrates a spiral displaced fracture through the humeral surgical neck (arrow). (B) Axillary radiograph of the humerus in a different patient demonstrates comminuted fractures of the humeral head and both tuberosities (arrows).

Key Facts

- Synonym: Broken arm, broken shoulder
- Definition: Disrupted humeral bone
- Classic imaging appearance
  - Linear lucency through proximal aspect of the humeral bone
  - Majority of proximal humeral fractures are non displaced
- Neer classification: Used to guide treatment and estimate the prognosis
  - The Neer classification system includes 4 segments
    - I: Greater tuberosity
    - II: Lesser tuberosity
    - III: Humeral head
    - IV: Humeral shaft
  - Also, Neer classification rates displacement
    - A fracture is displaced when there is more than 1 cm of displacement and 45° of angulation of any one fragment with respect to the others
  - One-part fractures are nondisplaced fractures
  - Two-part fractures involve any of the 4 parts and include 1 fragment that is displaced
    - Most common displacement: Medial and anterior displacement of the shaft in association with the fracture of the humeral neck
  - Three-part fractures include a displaced fracture of the surgical neck in addition to either a displaced greater tuberosity or lesser tuberosity fracture
  - Four-part fractures include displaced fractures of the surgical neck and both tuberosities

Proximal Humeral Fracture

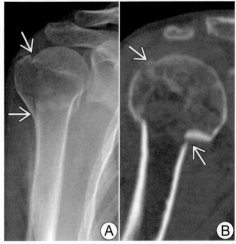

Proximal humeral fracture. (A) AP radiograph of the humerus shows nondisplaced fractures of the surgical neck and also the greater tuberosity (arrows). (B) CT scan with coronal reformatted image of the same patient confirms the nondisplaced fractures of the surgical neck and the greater tuberosity (arrows).

Imaging Findings

<u>General Features</u>
- Best imaging clue: Detection of fracture lucency
- Anatomy
  - Muscles: The supraspinatus and infraspinatus pull the greater tuberosity superiorly and the subscapularis pulls the lesser tuberosity medially, while the pectoralis major adducts the shaft medially

<u>Radiography Findings</u>
- AP view of the glenohumeral joint
  - Fracture displacements of the surgical neck
  - Fractures of the greater tuberosity when there is superior displacement
  - Fractures of the lesser tuberosity when there is medial displacement
- Scapular lateral
  - Anterior or posterior angulation of the surgical neck
  - Posterior displacement of the greater tuberosity fragment
- Axillary lateral
  - Tuberosity fragments
    - Anteromedial displacement of the lesser tuberosity
    - Postevolateval displacement of the greater tuberosity
  - Dislocation of the head can be identified

<u>CT Findings</u>
- Extent of tuberosity displacement
- Size of humeral head indentation fractures
- Amount of articular involvement in head-splitting fractures

<u>MR Findings</u>
- T1WI: Fractures seen as linear low signal areas
- T2WI
  - Fractures seen as linear high signal areas

Proximal Humeral Fracture

o Ligamentous and muscle injuries seen as areas of high signal edema

Imaging Recommendations
- Anteroposterior (AP) and axillary humerus and shoulder views are mandatory
- Axillary view with Velpeau bandage may be used for patients who cannot comply with the positioning required for an axillary view
- Angiogram: If a vascular injury is suspected

Differential Diagnosis
Shoulder Dislocation
- Humeral head is dislocated from the glenoid fossa
- May be associated with proximal humeral fracture
- In proximal humeral fracture without dislocation, the glenohumeral joint is intact

Pathology
General
- Etiology-Pathogenesis
  o Direct trauma to the arm or shoulder
  o Axial loading transmitted through the elbow
- Epidemiology
  o Proximal humeral fractures account for up to 5% of all fractures

Clinical Issues
Presentation
- Pain over the site of humeral fracture, deformity, ecchymosis, crepitus, limited range of motion
- Proximal humeral fractures are associated with neurovascular injuries
  o The axillary nerve is the most common nerve injured
Treatment
- Minimally displaced or nondisplaced: Conservatively
  o Immobilization with a sling and early range of motion exercises
- Two-part fractures: May reduce with glenohumeral reduction
- Three-part fractures: Open reduction and internal fixation
- Four-part fractures: Managed with hemiarthroplasty
Prognosis
- One-part fracture: Excellent
- Two and three-part fractures: Depending on the displaced fragments and associated early and late complications
- Four-part fractures: Up to 90% result in avascular necrosis of the humeral head

Selected References
1. Bernstein J et al: Evaluation of the Neer system of classification of proximal humeral fractures with computerized tomographic scans and plain radiographs. J Bone Joint Surg Am. 78:1371-1375, 1996
2. Lind T et al: The epidemiology of fractures of the proximal humerus. Arch. Orthop. Trauma Surg. 108:285, 1989
3. Neer CS et al: Displaced proximal humeral fractures. J. Bone Joint Surg. Am. 52:1077, 1970

Elbow Dislocation

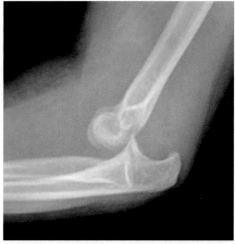

Lateral radiograph of elbow demonstrates a posterior dislocation. The ulna is displaced posteriorly by approximately one shaft width. No definite associated fractures are seen.

Key Facts
- Definition: Traumatic disarticulation of the elbow joint
- Classic imaging appearance
  - Posterior displacement of the ulna and radius
- Other key facts
  - Most commonly dislocates posteriorly (85-90%)
    - Other types include anterior, lateral, medial, and divergent
  - Associated with fractures up to 60% of the time
    - Coronoid process
    - Olecranon process
    - Medial epicondyle
    - Radial head
    - Articular surfaces
    - Distal radius and wrist fractures
  - Neurovascular injuries are uncommon
  - Radial head and ulna most often dislocate together in adults
    - Isolated radial head or ulnar dislocation more common in young children

Imaging Findings
<u>General Features</u>
- Disarticulation at the elbow joint
<u>Plain Film Findings (Elbow Series)</u>
- Usually obvious
- Associated fractures may be difficult to perceive
  - Fractures become more visible on post reduction views
  - Must identify entrapped fragments
    - Usually the medial epicondylar ossification center in children
    - Most often from a fracture of the coronoid process in adults

Elbow Dislocation

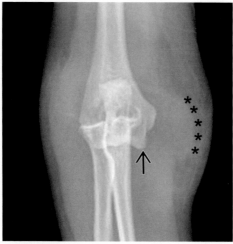

AP radiograph also demonstrates the posterior dislocation. Note the associated fracture (arrow) and large hemarthrosis (asterisks).

<u>CT Findings</u>
- Post reduction CT useful for defining fractures and entrapped fragments

<u>MR Findings</u>
- Useful for defining soft tissue injury
  - Ligamentous injury
  - Cartilage defects
    - Soft tissue injury may determine type of reconstruction and prognosis
- Aids with the diagnosis of subtle coronoid process fractures

<u>Imaging Recommendations</u>
- Standard 4 view elbow series
  - Post reduction views
- CT and MRI as needed to further define the extent of injury
- Angiography for suspected vascular injury

Differential Diagnosis
<u>Nursemaid's Elbow</u>
- Isolated dislocation of the radial head
  - Pediatric patients only
  - No dislocation of ulna

<u>Monteggia Fracture</u>
- Radial head dislocation with ulnar fracture

<u>Elbow Fractures Without Dislocation</u>
- No dislocation on plain films

Pathology
<u>General</u>
- Etiology-Pathogenesis
  - Hyperextension usually from a fall on an extended, abducted arm
    - Olecranon impinges on the olecranon fossa and forces the elbow apart

Elbow Dislocation

- - Collateral ligaments commonly avulse at their humeral attachments
- Epidemiology
  - o Third most common dislocation in adults
    - Shoulder and interphalangeal joints of fingers are first and second
    - More common in males
  - o Most common dislocation in children
  - o 50% from sports-related injuries

Staging or Grading Criteria

- Simpson
  - o Both radius and ulna
  - o Ulna alone
  - o Radius alone

Clinical Issues

Presentation

- Usually obvious
  - o Pain
  - o Limited range of motion
  - o When posterior
    - Elbow fixed with exaggerated prominence of the olecranon
  - o When anterior
    - Elbow held in full extension
  - o Hemarthrosis
  - o Pre and post reduction exam should evaluate for neurovascular injury

Natural History

- Often results in chronic instability
  - o Most commonly posterolateral instability
- Complications include
  - o Brachial artery injury
  - o Medial and ulnar nerve injury
  - o Myositis ossificans

Treatment

- Non-operative reduction and casting in cases without fracture
- Operative treatment
  - o Complex dislocations with associated fractures
  - o Severe instability with rupture of both medial collateral ligament and flexor forearm muscles

Prognosis

- 50% full recovery
- One third will have limited range of motion
  - o Usually less than 10 degrees
- Remaining 15% have more range of motion limitations

Selected References
1. Hildebrand KA et al: Acute elbow dislocations: simple and complex. Orthop Clin North Am. 30:63-79, 1999
2. Villarin LA et al: Emergency department evaluation and treatment of elbow and forearm injuries. Emerg Med Clin North Am. 17:843-58, 1999
3. Cohen MS et al: Acute elbow dislocation: evaluation and management. J Am Acad Orthop Surg. 6:15-23, 1998

Radial Head Fracture

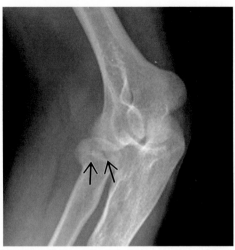

Radial head fracture. Oblique radiograph shows a comminuted fracture of radial head (arrows). The fracture extends to the articular surface.

Key Facts
- Synonym: Elbow fracture
- Classic imaging appearance
  - Minimally displaced fracture of radial head with hemarthrosis
    - Displacement of the posterior and/or anterior elbow fat pads
- Other key facts
  - Can be associated with injuries to the radial-ulnar interosseous membrane
  - Other associated fractures
    - Colles' fracture
    - Scaphoid fracture
    - Other distal radius, ulna, and carpal fractures
    - Radial capitellum fracture

Imaging Findings
General Features
- Best imaging clue: Displacement of the elbow fat pads on lateral plain film
- Fracture commonly located along lateral joint surface of radius
- Usually vertically oriented
- May see step off or abrupt angulation of radial head surface
- Disruption of the supinator fascial plane
CT Findings
- Useful in cases with severe comminution and elbow dislocation
MR Findings
- Greatly increases diagnostic sensitivity in indeterminate cases
- T1WI
  - Low signal intensity fracture line
- T2WI
  - Low signal intensity fracture line
  - Marrow edema
  - High signal intensity effusion

Radial Head Fracture

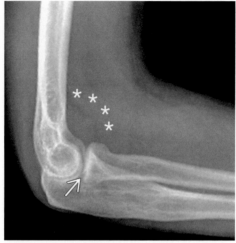

Radial head fracture. Lateral radiograph of elbow shows displacement of anterior fat pad, indicative of a large hemarthrosis (asterisks). Part of the intra-articular fracture is seen as subtle cortical irregularity (arrow).

- o Helpful in the exclusion of associated collateral ligament injury
  - ▪ May lead to instability

<u>Imaging Recommendations</u>
- Plain film
  - o AP, lateral, and oblique views
  - o Fractures may be occult on AP and lateral views
  - o Radial head view
    - ▪ Forearm in neutral rotation
    - ▪ Tube angled 45 degrees cephalad
- CT
  - o Comminuted fractures or indeterminate plain films
- MR
  - o Cases with high clinical suspicion and normal radiographs
  - o For evaluation of associated soft tissue injuries
- Radiographic examination of the wrist should be performed when radial head fractures are comminuted
  - o Essex-Lopresti fracture
    - ▪ Comminuted radial head fracture associated with radioulnar subluxation

Differential Diagnosis
<u>Radial Neck Fracture</u>
- More common in the pediatric population
  - o Radial neck fractured but radial head intact
  - o Fractures differentiated on imaging studies
<u>Distal Humerus Fracture</u>
- Fracture differentiated on imaging studies

Radial Head Fracture

Pathology
Genera
- Lack of radial head subchondral bone anterolaterally results in most fractures being located anterolaterally
- Etiology-Pathogenesis
  - Fall on an outstretched hand
    - Force is transmitted along the longitudinal axis of the radius
    - Radial head is compressed against the capitellum
- Epidemiology
  - Most common adult elbow injury
    - 50% of adult elbow injuries
    - 15% of elbow injuries in children
    - Supracondylar fractures more common in children

Classification
- Mason's classification of radial head fractures
  - Type 1 - less than 2 mm of displacement
  - Type 2 - minimally displaced with depression, angulation, and impaction
  - Type 3 - comminution of entire radial head

Clinical Issues
Presentation
- Tenderness to palpation over radial head
- Inability to pronate or supinate
- Crepitus with supination

Treatment
- Casting utilized in nondisplaced fractures
- For severely comminuted fractures the radial head may be excised

Prognosis
- Non-displaced fracture or successful early reduction results in minimal to no loss of elbow extension
- Displaced fracture or delayed management
  - Permanently restricted range of motion
  - Traumatic arthritis
  - Myositis ossificans

Selected References
1. Ring D et al: Mini-symposium: elbow problems, III: Elbow fractures in the adult. Current Orthopaedics. 11:242-48, 1997
2. Pitt MJ et al: Imaging of the elbow with an emphasis on trauma. Radiol Clin North Am. 28:293-305, 1990
3. Mason ML: Some observations on fractures of the head of the radius with a review of 100 cases. Br J Surg. 43:123-132, 1954

Monteggia Fracture

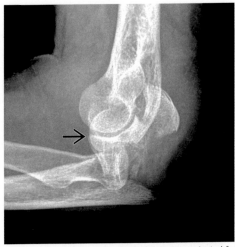

Monteggia fracture. Lateral view of the elbow shows a comminuted fracture of the ulna through the olecranon. The radial head is posteriorly dislocated from the capitellum (arrow).

Key Facts
- Synonym: Forearm fracture/dislocation
- Definition: Fracture of the ulna with dislocation of the radial head
- Classic imaging appearance
  - Proximal ulna fracture with anterior dislocation of the radial head

Imaging Findings
Plain Film Findings
- Fracture through the proximal or middle third of the ulna
- Radial head dislocation
  - Dislocation may by subtle
  - Dislocation may be anterior or posterior
  - The long axis of the radius should line up with the capitellum in all projections (radial-capitellar line)
- The direction of the radial head dislocation is usually oriented in the same direction as the apex of the ulnar fracture
- Ulnar fracture is usually transverse or slightly oblique, comminution is unusual
CT Findings
- Post reduction CT useful for defining fractures and entrapped fragments
MR Findings
- Useful for defining soft tissue injury
  - Ligamentous injury
  - Cartilage defects
Imaging Recommendations
- AP and lateral forearm series
- Four view elbow series
  - Radial head dislocation may not be apparent on AP and lateral forearm films

Monteggia Fracture

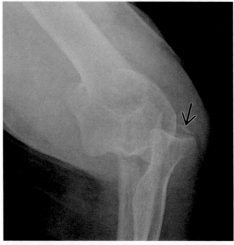

Monteggia fracture. Oblique film of elbow shows posterior dislocation of radial head. Indicates a capitellum fracture fragment (arrow).

Differential Diagnosis
Galeazzi Fracture
- Distal radius fracture with dislocation of the distal radioulnar joint

Nightstick Fracture
- Isolated fracture of the ulna without radial head dislocation

Pathology
General
- Etiology-Pathogenesis
  - Most commonly occurs from fall on an outstretched arm with forced pronation
  - A direct blow to the forearm may also produce the injury
  - When the ulna is fractured the force is transmitted along the interosseous membrane displacing the proximal radius
- Epidemiology
  - 1-2% of all forearm fractures

Classification
- Bado
  - Type I - fracture of the proximal or middle third of the ulna with anterior dislocation of the radial head
  - Type II - fracture of the proximal or middle third of the ulna with posterior dislocation of the radial head
  - Type III - fracture of the ulnar metaphysis with lateral dislocation of the radial head
  - Type IV - fracture of the proximal or middle third of the ulna and radius with anterior dislocation of the radial head

Clinical Issues
Presentation
- Elbow pain, swelling, deformity

Monteggia Fracture

- Crepitus at the elbow
- Limited flexion and rotation at the elbow joint

Natural History
- Complications
  - Radial nerve injury
  - Malunion or nonunion
  - Recurrent dislocation of radial head
  - Radioulnar synostosis

Treatment
- Closed Monteggia fracture in adults
  - Radial head dislocation should be reduce emergently followed by elective internal fixation of the ulna fracture
- Closed Monteggia fracture in children
  - Closed reduction with casting
- Open fracture dislocation
  - Requires open reduction internal fixation in all patients

Prognosis
- Generally good prognosis with timely diagnosis, adequate reduction, and stable fixation

Selected References
1. Perron AD et al: Orthopedic pitfalls in the ED: Galeazzi and Monteggia fracture-dislocation. Am J Emerg Med. 19:225-8, 2001
2. Ring D et al: Monteggia fractures in children and adults. J Am Acad Orthop Surg. 6:215-24, 1998
3. Ring D et al: Monteggia fractures in adults. J Bone Joint Surg Am. 80:1733-44, 1998

Colles' Fracture

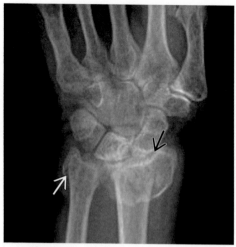

Colles' fracture. AP wrist film shows a transverse, comminuted, and impacted fracture of the distal radius. Note the extension into the radiocarpal joint (black arrow). There is an associated fracture of the ulnar styloid (white arrow).

Key Facts
- Synonym(s): Wrist fracture, distal radius and ulna fracture
- Definition: Transverse distal radius fracture with dorsal displacement, angulation, and impaction
- Classic imaging appearance
  - Transverse fracture or the distal radius
  - Approximately 2.5 cm from the articular surface
  - Dorsally angulated
  - Dorsally displaced
  - Dorsally impacted
  - Associated with ulnar styloid fracture
- Other key facts
  - Most common fracture of the forearm
  - Originally described prior to discovery of x-rays
    - Original description did not include precise anatomical detail provided by the radiograph
  - Often associated with other fractures in the elderly
    - Radial head fractures
    - 9% of proximal humerus fractures associated with distal radius fractures
    - 8% of hip fractures associated with distal radius fractures

Imaging Findings
General Features
- Transverse distal radius fracture
- Often comminuted
- 70% extend to radiocarpal and/or radioulnar joint
  - 35% involve both
  - Fragmentation of the articular surface of the radius is common
    - Fragmentation most pronounced dorsally

Colles' Fracture

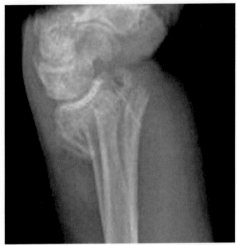

Colles' fracture. Lateral view of the wrist demonstrates dorsal angulation and displacement. The degree of impaction is well shown.

- Impacted
  - Degree of impaction is greater on the lateral and dorsal radius
- 60% have an associated ulnar styloid fracture
  - Less commonly associated fracture of the head or neck of the ulna

CT Findings
- Indicated for question intra-articular extension
- Used for operative planning
- Evaluation of uncertain radiographic findings

MR Findings
- Used to evaluate associated injures
  - Median nerve in acute carpal tunnel syndrome
  - Triangular fibrocartilage tears
    - Associated in 40-78% of distal radius fractures
  - Carpal ligament injures
    - Associated in 50% of distal radius fractures

Imaging Recommendations
- Standard 4 view wrist series
- Must consider imaging workup of other potential injuries
  - Proximal humerus fracture
  - Hip fracture
  - Carpal fracture/dislocations
  - Soft tissue injury

Differential Diagnosis

Other Distal Radius and Ulna Fractures
- Reverse Colles', Smith's fracture, Barton's fracture, chauffeur's fracture, Hutchinson's fracture
- Differentiated on imaging studies

Carpal Bone Fractures
- Differentiated on imaging studies

Colles' Fracture

Pathology
General
- Etiology-Pathogenesis
  - Fall on an outstretched hand
  - Dorsal surface of radius is compressed
    - Results in comminution of posterior cortex
  - Anterior surface is placed under tension
    - Results in dorsal angulation or displacement of anterior cortex
- Epidemiology
  - Most often occurs in older persons
    - More often in post menopausal females
    - By age 60 is 6 times more common in females
  - In young adults due to motor vehicle and motorcycle collisions
    - High impact forces create more complex fractures
    - Often associated with fracture dislocation of the carpus

Classification
- Modified Frykman
  - Extra-articular fracture of the distal radius
  - Extra-articular fracture of the distal radius with a fracture of the ulnar styloid
  - Intra-articular fracture of the radiocarpal joint
  - Intra-articular fracture of the radiocarpal joint with a fracture of the ulnar styloid
  - Comminuted intra-articular fracture of the radiocarpal and radioulnar joints
  - Comminuted intra-articular fracture of the radiocarpal and radioulnar joints with an ulnar styloid fracture

Clinical Issues
Presentation
- Pain, swelling, posterior angulation of the wrist

Natural History
- Pain
- Loss of range of motion; strength
- Progression of deformity once cast is removed
- Occasional acute carpal tunnel syndrome
- Occasional reflex sympathetic dystrophy

Treatment
- Closed reduction with casting and restoration of the length of the radius
- Open fixation
  - When casting fails to maintain alignment
  - Greater than 2 mm of articular step off
  - Acute carpal tunnel syndrome

Prognosis
- Poor prognosis with significant morbidity in up to 50% of cases

Selected References
1. Ritchie JV et al: Emergency department evaluation and treatment of wrist injuries. Emerg Med Clin North Am. 17:823-42, 1999
2. Eustace S et al: Emergency MR imaging of orthopedic trauma. Current and future directions. Radiol Clin North Am. 37:975-94, 1999
3. Spence LD et al: MRI of fractures of the distal radius: Comparison with conventional radiographs. Skeletal Radiol. 27:244-9, 1998

Scaphoid Fracture

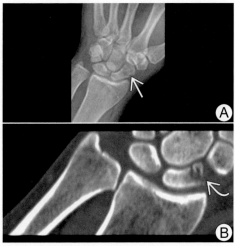

Scaphoid fracture. (A) AP view of the wrist shows fracture through waist of scaphoid (arrow). Scaphoid fracture (B) coronal reformatted CT through the radial carpal joint confirms fracture of waist of scaphoid (curved arrow).

Key Facts
- Synonym: Carpo-navicular fracture
- Definition: Traumatic injury to the scaphoid
- Classic imaging appearance
  - Characteristically minimally displaced fracture
  - Fine transverse or slightly oblique lucent fracture line
- Other key facts
  - Most commonly fractured carpal bone
  - Usually from fall on an outstretched, dorsiflexed hand
  - Most commonly seen in young adults
  - May lead to nonunion and avascular necrosis of proximal fragment
    - Arterial supply enters distally
    - Blood supply to proximal fragment disrupted with fracture

Imaging Findings
General Features
- Diagnosis made from the AP wrist view
  - Fractures of scaphoid tuberosity may only be seen on oblique and lateral views
  - Fractures of scaphoid waist are better demonstrated on the oblique projection
  - Fractures of proximal pole are clearly seen on the AP view
- Most fractures run transversely or slightly oblique to the long axis of scaphoid

CT Findings
- May demonstrate radiographically occult fractures
- Multidetector CT allows for high resolution coronal and sagittal reformations relative to the axis of the scaphoid

MR Findings
- T1WI give anatomic information

Scaphoid Fracture

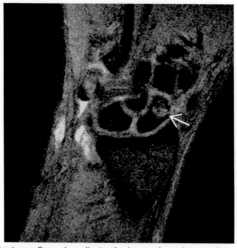

Scaphoid fracture. Coronal gradient echo image shows increased signal intensity (arrow) within scaphoid consistent with marrow edema.

- o The fracture line itself is seen as a low signal intensity line
- o Low signal throughout the scaphoid represents marrow edema
- STIR rapidly performed and very sensitive
  - o Absence of high signal excludes a fracture
  - o When edema is present the fracture is anatomically confirmed with T1WI

Bone Scintigraphy Findings
- May assist diagnosis of scaphoid fracture
  - o Scan may not be positive for 48 hours to 1 week
- Radioisotope uptake in overlying soft tissues may lead to false positive studies

Imaging Recommendations
- Radiographic series consists of 4 views
  - o AP
  - o Lateral
  - o 45 degree oblique
  - o AP with ulnar deviation (scaphoid view)
- MDCT
  - o 1.25 mm axial images
    - Soft tissue and bone algorithm
  - o Sagittal and coronal reformations relative to long axis of scaphoid
- MRI
  - o Trauma screening
    - Coronal TI
    - Coronal STIR

Differential Diagnosis
Soft Tissue Injury Without Fracture
- Imaging examinations rule out fracture
Psuedofracture
- Margins of the trabeculae in bone may be mistaken for fracture

- Prominent tubercle along radial margin of the waist can be mistaken for fracture

Pathology

General
- Etiology-Pathogenesis
  - Fall on an outstretched dorsiflexed hand
    - Angulation between the proximal and distal carpal rows places great stress on the narrow scaphoid waist
- Epidemiology
  - Most commonly between ages of 15 and 40 years
    - Fractures in young children are rare
    - Sharp decline in the incidence after 40
    - Rarely encountered after 60

Staging Criteria
- Modified Herbert Staging
  - Acute stable
  - Acute unstable
  - Delayed Union
  - Established Nonunion

Clinical Issues

Presentation
- Pain in the anatomic snuffbox
  - High negative predictive value
  - Only 50-60% positive predictive value

Natural History
- Delayed and nonunion 5-10%
- Avascular necrosis up to 30%

Treatment
- Casting for stable injuries
- Screw fixation and/or bone grafting for unstable injuries

Prognosis
- Depends on location of fracture and time to diagnosis
  - Better prognosis for more distal fractures and early diagnosis

Selected References
1. Eustace, S et al: MR Imaging of acute orthopedic trauma to the extremities. Radiol. Clin. North Am. 35:615, 1997
2. Hunter, JC et al: MR imaging of clinically suspected scaphoid fractures. A.J.R. 168:1287, 1997
3. Hindman, BW et al: Occult fractures of the carpals and metacarpals: Demonstration by CT. A.J.R. 153:529, 1989

First Metacarpal Fracture

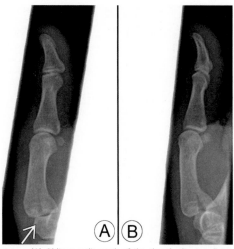

Bennett fracture. (A) Oblique radiograph of the thumb shows a Bennett fracture. Injury is oriented with long axis of the digit at base of first metacarpal (arrow). (B) Lateral radiograph shows dorsal and radial displacement characteristic of a Bennett fracture.

Key Facts
- Synonym(s): Bennett fracture versus Rolando fracture
- Definition: Intra-articular first metacarpal fracture
  - Bennett - single intra-articular fracture with dorsal, radial dislocation
  - Rolando - three part intra-artricular fracture at the trapeziometacarpal joint
- Classic imaging appearance
  - Lucency at the base of the first metacarpal
- Other key facts regarding both fractures
  - Must be distinguished between extra-articular fractures located distal to the metacarpal-phalyngeal (MCP) joint
    - Usually more transverse
    - Located at the proximal metaphseal-diaphyseal junction
    - More conservatively managed

Imaging Findings
<u>General Features</u>
- Bennett
  - Intra-articular fracture/dislocation of the base of the first metacarpal
    - Oblique fracture line with a triangular fragment at ulnar base of metacarpal
  - Small anterior fragment of metacarpal maintains alignment with trapezium
    - Held in place by the anterior oblique ligament's attachment to the trapezium
  - Dorsal and radial dislocation secondary to continued force from abductor pollicus longus
- Rolando

First Metacarpal Fracture

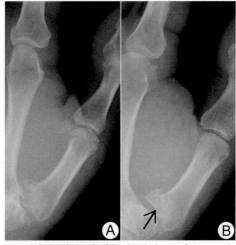

Rolando fracture. (A) AP radiograph of the thumb shows a fracture at the base of the first metacarpal. (B) Shows the intra-articular extension (arrow).

- o Configuration of a T or Y
- o Both volar and dorsal fragments present
  - Volar carpal ligament remains attached to the volar fragment
  - Adductor pollicus longus tendon remains attached to the dorsal fragment

CT Findings
- May help define the degree of comminution and subluxation

MR Findings
- Useful for evaluating for associated tendonous and ligamentous injury

Imaging Recommendations
- Standard AP, lateral, and oblique radiographs of the hand
- Traction may be needed to assess the degree of comminution in Rolando fractures
- CT to further define the injury as needed
- MRI to assess for soft tissue injury

Differential Diagnosis

Extra-Articular First Metacarpal Fracture
- More proximally located and transversely oriented
- Usually heals with closed reduction

Comminuted First Metacarpal Fracture
- Greater than three part fracture
- Pilon type fracture with articular surface impaction

First Carpometacarpal Dislocation
- Rarely occurs without associated fracture

Pathology

General
- Etiology-Pathogenesis
  - o Axial loading of a partially flexed first metacarpal
    - Common injury from punching

First Metacarpal Fracture

- Epidemiology
  - Bennett
    - Most frequent first metacarpal fracture
  - Rolando
    - Uncommon first metacarpal fracture

Classification
- Intra-articular first metacarpal fracture
  - Bennett
  - Rolando
- Extra-articular first metacarpal fracture
  - Transverse
  - Oblique
  - Epiphyseal

Clinical Issues
Presentation
- Patients present with swelling and pain at the base of the thumb
- On examination motion is limited and carpal metacarpal instability is frequent

Natural History
- Must be recognized and treated to prevent severe osteoarthritis, loss of mobility, and pain

Treatment
- Closed reduction and thumb spica cast immobilization may be effective in some cases
  - Small avulsion fractures
  - Less than 1 mm of articular incongruity
  - Minimal instability
    - Must monitor closed reduction with serial radiography
- Internal fixation frequently required
  - Subluxation
    - Force of abductor pollicus longus leads to dorsal and radial displacement
  - More than 1 mm of articular incongruity is an operative indication
  - Unstable fracture

Prognosis
- Closely related to the complexity of the original injury
  - Good prognosis
    - Stable fractures
    - Simple fracture pattern
    - Limited ligamentous injury
  - Poor prognosis
    - Comminution (Rolando)
    - Articular surface damage
    - Ligamentous injury
    - Unstable fractures

Selected References
1. Soyer AD: Fractures of the base of the first metacarpal: Current treatment options. J Am Acad Orthop Surg. 6:403-12, 1999
2. Kahler DM: Fractures and dislocations of the base of the thumb. J South Orthop Assoc. 4:69-76, 1995
3. Bennet EH: Fractures of the metacarpal bones. Dublin Med Sci J. 73:72-75, 1882

Phalangeal Fracture of the Hand

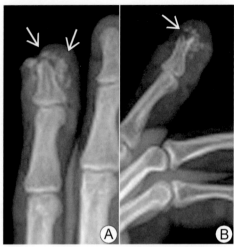

Phalangeal fracture. (A) Oblique, and (B) Lateral views of the second digit show comminuted displaced fracture of the distal phalanx with laceration of the overlying soft tissue (arrows).

Key Facts
- Synonym: Finger fracture, broken finger, finger jam, jammed finger
- Definition: Discontinuation of the cortex of one of the finger bones
- Classic imaging appearance: Fracture lucency through the fractured bone
- Associated with
  - Laceration of the soft tissues
  - Ligamentous injuries
- Classification
  - Proximal phalanx
    - Collateral ligament avulsion fracture (gamekeeper's thumb)
    - Proximal phalanx base fracture with dorsal angulation
    - Proximal interphalangeal joint dorsal fracture-dislocations
  - Middle phalanx
    - Oblique or transverse shaft fractures
    - Avulsion fracture of the base of the middle phalanx at the proximal interphalangeal joint (volar plate fracture)
  - Distal phalanx
    - Tuberosity fractures
    - Interphalangeal joint fracture-dislocations (mallet finger)

Imaging Findings
General Features
- Best imaging clue: Detection of fracture lucency through the fractured bone
Radiography Findings
- AP view of the injured finger
  - Comminuted fracture of the tuberosity of the distal phalanx
- True lateral of the injured finger without overlapping
  - Mallet finger and also volar plate injuries
- Oblique view of the injured finger

Phalangeal Fracture of the Hand

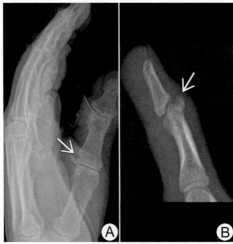

Phalangeal fracture. (A) Oblique radiograph of the first digit shows avulsion fracture at the base of the first proximal phalanx (gamekeeper's thumb) (arrow). (B) Lateral radiograph of the second digit shows avulsion fracture at the dorsal aspect of the distal phalanx with soft tissue swelling (mallet finger) (arrow).

- o Avulsion fractures of the collateral ligaments

CT Findings
- Not performed routinely
- Definition of the extent of intraarticular involvement

MR Findings
- Not performed routinely
- Evaluation of injured ligaments
  - o T1W: Anatomic location
  - o T2W: High signal within areas injured

Imaging Recommendations
- Usually plain radiographs are sufficient for diagnosing phalangeal fractures
- Stress views if no fracture identified on routine views, but fracture clinically suspected
- CT maybe used in preoperative planning and assessment of displaced fragments
  - o 1 mm axial images
  - o Sagittal and coronal reformations
  - o Bone and soft tissue algorithms
- MRI in acute trauma screening
  - o Not performed routinely
  - o STIR and T1W sequences

Differential Diagnosis
Ligamentous Injuries
- May mimic clinical presentation of fractures
- Plain radiographs aid in detecting underlying fracture

Phalangeal Fracture of the Hand

Pathology

General

- Etiology-Pathogenesis
  - o Proximal interphalangeal joint fracture
    - Axial blow to the finger
    - Rotational hyperextension injury
  - o Middle phalanx: Hyperextension avulsion injury at the palmar aspect of the base of the middle phalanx (volar plate fracture)
  - o Distal phalanx
    - Tuberosity: Crush injury
    - Avulsion at the base of the distal phalanx: Blow to the end of an extended finger
- Epidemiology
  - o Most common fractured finger bone is the distal phalanx
  - o Up to 10% of all fractures

Staging or Grading Criteria

- Dependent on location, fracture orientation, and degree of initial displacement
  - o Stable fractures
    - Tuberosity fractures, nondisplaced fractures with intact cortex
  - o Non-stable fractures
    - Interphalangeal unicondylar or bicondylar fractures
    - Diaphyseal displaced fractures of the proximal and middle phalanges

Clinical Issues

Presentation

- Swelling, ecchymosis, and decreased range of motion, deformity

Natural History

- Limited range of motion
- Premature osteoarthritic changes
- Deformity

Treatment

- Management of the associated soft tissue injury
- Non displaced, stable fractures
  - o Closed reduction with splinting
  - o Early rehabilitation
- Displaced fractures
  - o Percutaneous pinning
- Complex phalangeal fractures
  - o Mini-fragment screws and plates

Prognosis

- Excellent if detected early with appropriate treatment
- Proximal phalangeal fractures may disrupt or adhese the extensor or flexor mechanisms with loss of motility of the fingers

Selected References

1. Lubahn JD et al: Fractures of the distal interphalangeal joint. Clin. Orthop. 327:12-20, 1996
2. Gonzalez MH et al: Intramedullary nailing of proximal phalangeal fractures. J Hand Surg. 20(5):808-12, 1995
3. Weiss AP et al: Distal unicondylar fractures of the proximal phalanx. J Hand Surg [Am]. 18(4):594, 1993

PocketRadiologist®
ER-Trauma
Top 100 Diagnoses

PELVIC FRACTURES

Sacral Fracture

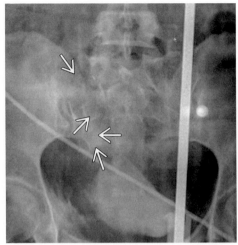

Sacral Fracture. Coned down AP radiograph of the pelvis obtained on the trauma board demonstrates disruption of the arcuate lines (arrows), indicating a vertical fracture. Note: The contralateral arcuate lines are normal.

Key Facts
- Synonym: Broken sacrum
- Definition: Disruption of the sacral bone
- Most sacral fractures are associated with pelvic or lumbar spine fractures
  - Less than 5% of sacral fractures involve only the sacrum
- Classification
  - Vertical: Part of complex pelvic fractures, 90% of cases
  - Transverse: Result of direct applied forces, through the sacral ala or sacral arcades up to 8% of cases
    - U-shaped fractures: Variation of transverse fracture, result of axial loading, bilateral transforaminal fractures

Imaging Findings
<u>General Features</u>
- Best imaging clue
  - Identifying the lucent fracture line
  - Disruption of the sacral arcuate lines
- Other generic features
  - Presence of a presacral hematoma provides secondary evidence for an acute sacral fracture
  - Transverse injuries may have fracture lines parallel to the scanning plane and be missed
  - Isolated fractures are usually transverse
    - High transverse (S1 or S2) fractures are due to high energy injury such as fall
    - Low transverse (S3 or S4) fractures due to direct blow
- Anatomy: Sacral body, sacral alae, paired sacral foramina
<u>Radiographic Findings</u>
- AP pelvis: Disruption of curved lines on the superior margin of the sacral foramina suggests the presence of vertical fractures

Sacral Fracture

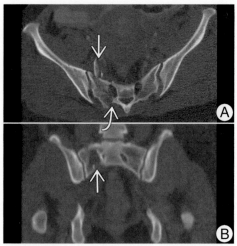

Sacral Fracture. (A) Initial axial CT scan through the pelvis shows a comminuted fracture fragment displaced anteriorly (arrow). Note the disrupted foramina (curved arrow). (B) CT scan of same patient with coronal reformats demonstrates the vertical fracture (arrow).

- Lateral pelvis: Overriding and displacement of the fracture fragment
- Pelvic inlet: Fractures of the anterior sacral foramina
- Pelvic outlet: Fractures of the sacral body, sacral wings including all the sacral foraminal lines

CT Findings
- Coronal: Vertical fractures
- Sagittal: High transverse fractures show overriding
- Axial: Oblique and vertical fractures

MR Findings
- T1W: Fracture appears as linear areas of low signal
- T2W: Fracture appears as linear areas of high signal with surrounding high signal edema

Imaging Recommendations
- Pelvic plain films should be the initial imaging method
  o Tailor the exam to the patient's condition
- CT indications
  o More detailed depiction of the fracture orientation
  o Extent of involvement of the foramina
  o Evaluation of associated injuries
- MRI is indicated for radiographically occult fractures with a high clinical suspicion

Pathology
- None relevant to this case

Differential Diagnosis
Sacral Insufficiency Fracture
- Occur from physiologic stress on bone weakened by osteoporosis of variant etiologies

Sacral Fracture

- Pathognomonic appearance confined to the sacral ala (Honda sign), juxta-articular and vertical

Clinical Issues
<u>Presentation</u>
- Sacral tenderness and vague to specific neurological symptoms
<u>Treatment</u>
- Dependent on stability
  o Conservative if stable
  o Reduction and fixation if unstable
<u>Prognosis</u>
- Variable and dependent on neurological deficits

Selected References
1. Carter TR et al: Pubic diastases with longitudinal fracture of the sacral body: Case report. J. Trauma. 30:627, 1990
2. Denis F et al: Sacral fractures: An important problem. Retrospective analysis of 236 cases. Clin. Orthop. 227:67, 1988
3. Jackson H et al: The sacral arcuate lines in upper sacral fractures. Radiology. 145:35, 1982

Vertical Shear Pelvic Injury

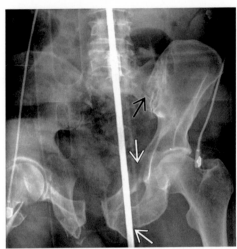

Vertical shear pelvic fracture. AP pelvic radiograph. Fractures of left superior & inferior pubic rami (white arrows). Fracture of sacral ala (black arrow). Widening of symphysis pubis is apparent. Vertical displacement of left hemipelvis differentiates this injury from the anterior compression fracture.

Key Facts
- Synonym: Malgaigne fracture
- Definition: Unstable pelvic fracture from an axial load to one side of the pelvis
- Classic imaging appearance
  - Vertically displaced hemipelvis
- Other key facts
  - Usually results from a fall or motor vehicle collision
  - Concomitant injuries are frequent because of force required to produce this fracture may result in other injuries
    - Traumatic brain injury 51%
    - Long bone fracture 48%
    - Thoracic injury 20%
    - Urethral injury in males 15%
    - Intra-abdominal organ injury 7-10%

Imaging Findings
General Features
- Anterior pelvis
  - Fractures of the superior and inferior pubic rami
- Posterior pelvis
  - Vertical fracture of the ipsilateral sacral ala
- Differentiated from an anterior compression fracture by the vertical displacement of the hemipelvis
Radiography Findings
- AP radiograph as part of the trauma series directs the need for further views

Vertical Shear Pelvic Injury

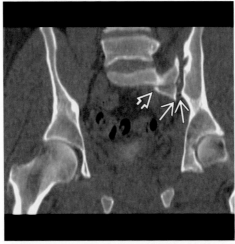

Vertical shear pelvic fracture. Coronal reformatted CT scan through left sacroiliac joint demonstrates diastasis of sacroiliac joint, vertical displacement of hemipelvis (arrows), and fracture of sacral ala (open arrow).

- Pelvic inlet view
  - Allows for visualization of AP displacement, internal/external rotation, and sacral impaction
- Pelvic outlet view
  - Demonstrates vertical displacement
  - Allows evaluation of the sacral foramina

CT Findings
- CT allows for better detection and definition of the complex spatial relationships of pelvic ring fractures
- Simultaneous evaluation of associated abdominal and pelvic injuries
  - Pelvic hemorrhage
  - Bladder injury
  - Solid organ injury

MR Findings
- Not used routinely in the evaluation of pelvic ring fractures

Angiography Findings
- Embolization may be indicated to treat life threatening pelvic hemorrhage

Imaging Recommendations
- Pelvis plain films
- Thin section CT with sagittal, coronal, and 3D reformations
- CT cystogram in pelvic ring fractures or with patients with hematuria
- Retrograde urethrogram in males with bleeding from the meatus

Differential Diagnosis

Acetabular Fracture
- Differentiated by imaging studies

Pelvic Insuffiency Fractures
- Elderly patients
- Less forceful mechanism of injury

Vertical Shear Pelvic Injury

Other Pelvic Ring Fractures
- Differentiated by imaging studies

Pathology
General
- Etiology-Pathogenesis
  o Mechanism created by a forceful vector from the femur to the ipsilateral hemipelvis
- Epidemiology
  o 6-16% of pelvic ring fractures
Classification of Pelvic Ring Fractures
- Vertical shear pelvic fracture
- Lateral compression pelvic fracture
- Anterior compression pelvic fracture

Clinical Issues
Presentation
- Pelvic pain
- Pelvic instability
- Foreshortened ipsilateral lower extremity due to vertical elevation of hemipelvis
Natural History
- Overall mortality in pelvic ring fractures is approximately 6%
  o Pelvic hemorrhage 39%
  o Traumatic brain injury 31%
  o Multiple organ failure 30%
- Immediate complications
  o Pelvic hemorrhage in up to 75% of patients
  o Bladder injury
    ▪ Extraperitoneal rupture due to pelvic fracture fragments
  o Urethral injury from shearing forces of the disrupted pelvic ring
  o Nerve injury
    ▪ Sacral plexus
    ▪ Sacral nerve roots
    ▪ Sciatic nerve
- Early and late complications
  o Thromboembolic disease; pain; malunion; osteoarthritis
Treatment
- Immediate stabilization with external fixator devices to decrease hemorrhage
- Embolization for uncontrollable hemorrhage
- Open reduction and internal fixation
Prognosis
- Related to residual deformity after treatment
  o Little to no residual deformity
    ▪ 12-18% morbidity
  o Residual deformity
    ▪ Up to 70% morbidity

Selected References
1. Hunter JC et al: Pelvic and acetabular trauma. Radiol Clin North Am. 35: 559-90, 1997
2. McCort JJ et al: Bladder injury and pelvic fractures. Emerg Radiol. 1:47-51, 1994
3. Burgess AR et al: Pelvic ring disruptions: Effective classification system and treatment protocols. J Trauma. 30:848-56, 1990

Lateral Pelvic Compression Fract.

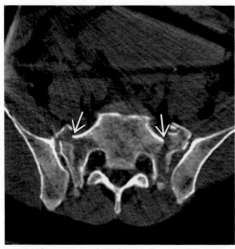

Lateral compression fracture. Axial CT through the sacroiliac joints show bilateral comminuted sacral ala fractures (arrows).

Key Facts
- Synonym: Lateral pelvic ring fracture
- Definition: Pelvic fracture secondary to a high energy lateral force to the pelvis
- Classic imaging appearance
  - Bilateral, superior and inferior pubic rami fractures with bilateral sacral ala fractures
- Other key facts
  - Most common pelvic ring fracture
  - Associated vascular injury is less common than in other types of pelvic ring fractures
  - Concomitant injuries are frequent because of forceful mechanism of injury required to produce this fracture
    - Traumatic brain injury 51%
    - Long bone fracture 48%
    - Thoracic injury 20%
    - Urethral injury in males 15%
    - Intra-abdominal organ injury 7-10%

Imaging Findings
<u>General Features</u>
- Sacral buckle fractures
  - Vertically oriented sacral fractures
- Superior and inferior pubic rami fractures, often horizontal in orientation
- Overlap pubic rami fracture fragments
- Iliac wing fractures may also be present
- Internal rotation of hemipelvis on the affected side
<u>Radiography Findings</u>
- Radiographic findings may be subtle
  - Slight cortical disruption of the sacral promontory and neural foramina

Lateral Pelvic Compression Fract.

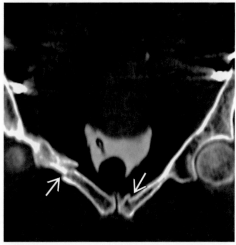

Lateral compression fracture. Coronal reformation through the symphysis pubis shows bilateral superior pubic rami fractures (arrows). The fragments of both fractures characteristically overlap. Artifacts are noted from the external fixator applied in the trauma room prior to CT.

- AP radiograph as part of the trauma series directs the need for further views
- Pelvic inlet view
  - Allows for visualization of AP displacement, internal/external rotation, and sacral impaction
- Pelvic outlet view
  - Demonstrates vertical displacement
  - Allows evaluation of the sacral foramina

CT Findings
- CT allows for better detection and definition of the complex spatial relationships of pelvic ring fractures
- Simultaneous evaluation of associated abdominal and pelvic injuries
  - Pelvic hemorrhage; bladder injury; solid organ injury

MR Findings
- Not used routinely in the evaluation of pelvic ring fractures

Angiography Findings
- Embolization may be indicated to treat life threatening pelvic hemorrhage

Imaging Recommendations
- Pelvis plain films
- Thin section CT with sagittal, coronal, and 3D reformations
- CT cystogram in pelvic ring fractures or with patients with gross hematuria
- Retrograde urethrogram in males with bleeding from the meatus

Differential Diagnosis
Acetabular Fracture
- Differentiated by imaging studies

Lateral Pelvic Compression Fract.

Pelvic Insufficiency Fractures
- Elderly patients; less forceful mechanism of injury

Other Pelvic Ring Fractures
- Differentiated by imaging studies

Pathology
General
- Etiology-Pathogenesis
  - Side-impact motor vehicle collisions and pedestrians struck by motor vehicles from the side
- Epidemiology
  - 57-71% of pelvic ring fractures

Classification of Pelvic Ring Fractures
- Vertical shear pelvic fracture
- Lateral compression pelvic fracture
- Anterior compression pelvic fracture

Clinical Issues
Presentation
- Pelvic pain; pelvic instability; internally rotated hemipelvis

Natural History
- Overall mortality in pelvic ring fractures is approximately 6%
  - Pelvic hemorrhage 39%
  - Traumatic brain injury 31%
  - Multiple organ failure 30%
- Immediate complications
  - Pelvic hemorrhage in up to 75% of patients
  - Bladder injury
    - Extraperitoneal rupture due to pelvic fracture fragments
    - Intraperitoneal rupture less commonly associated with pelvic ring fracture
  - Urethral injury from shearing forces of the disrupted pelvic ring
  - Nerve injury
    - Sacral plexus; sacral nerve roots; sciatic nerve
- Early and late complications
  - Thromboembolic disease; pain; malunion; osteoarthritis

Treatment
- Immediate stabilization with external fixator devices to decrease hemorrhage
- Embolization for uncontrollable hemorrhage
- Open reduction and internal fixation

Treatment
- Immediate stabilization with external fixator devices to decrease hemorrhage
- Embolization for uncontrollable hemorrhage
- Open reduction and internal fixation

Prognosis
- Related to residual deformity after treatment

Selected References
1.   Young JW: Pelvic injuries. Semin Musculoskelet Radiol. 2:83-104, 1998
2.   Resnik CS et al: Diagnosis of pelvic fractures in patients with acute pelvic trauma: efficacy of plain radiographs. AJR Am J Roentgenol. 158:109-12, 1992
3.   Tile M: Pelvic ring fractures: should they be fixed? J Bone Joint Surg Br. 70 :1-12, 1988

Anterior Compression Fracture

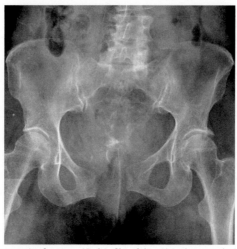

Anterior compression fracture. AP plain film of the pelvis shows marked diastasis of the symphysis pubis.

Key Facts
- Synonym: Anterior pelvic ring fracture
- Definition: Disruption of the bony structure of the pelvis secondary to an anterior or posterior force to the superior pelvis
- Classic imaging appearance
  - Diastasis of the symphysis pubis
  - Longitudinal fractures of the rami
- Other key facts
- Concomitant injuries are frequent because of forceful mechanism of injury
  - Traumatic brain injury 51%
  - Long bone fracture 48%
  - Thoracic injury 20%
  - Urethral injury in males 15%
  - Intra-abdominal organ injury 7-10%

Imaging Findings
General Features
- Pubic diastasis (> 1 cm) with or without sacroiliac joint disruption
- Unilateral or bilateral external rotation of the hemipelvis
- Vertically oriented pubic rami fractures
- Disruption of one or both sacroiliac joints
Radiography Findings
- AP radiograph as part of the trauma series directs the need for further views
- Pelvic inlet view
  - Allows for visualization of AP displacement, internal/external rotation, and sacral impaction
- Pelvic outlet view
  - Demonstrates vertical displacement
  - Allows evaluation of the sacral foramina

Anterior Compression Fracture

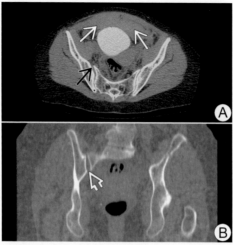

Anterior compression fracture. (A) Axial pelvic CT shows widening of right sacroiliac joint (black arrow) and associated hemorrhage from pubic rami fractures in pre vesical space (white arrows). There is no bladder rupture. (B) Coronal reformation shows widening of right sacroiliac joint (open arrow).

CT Findings
- CT allows for better detection and definition of the complex spatial relationships of pelvic ring fractures
- Simultaneous evaluation of associated abdominal and pelvic injuries
  - Pelvic hemorrhage; bladder injury; solid organ injury

MR Findings
- Not used routinely in the evaluation of pelvic ring fractures

Angiography Findings
- Embolization may be indicated to treat life threatening pelvic hemorrhage

Imaging Recommendations
- Pelvic plain films
- Thin section CT with sagittal, coronal, and 3D reformations
- CT cystogram in pelvic ring fractures or with patients with gross hematuria
- Retrograde urethrogram in males with bleeding from meatus

Differential Diagnosis

Acetabular Fracture
- Differentiated by imaging studies

Pelvic Insufficiency Fractures
- Elderly patients
- Less forceful mechanism of injury

Other Pelvic Ring Fractures
- Differentiated by imaging studies

Pathology

General
- Etiology-Pathogenesis
  - Caused by a forceful blow to the anterior or posterior pelvis

- Most occur from frontal deceleration motor vehicle collisions
- Motorcycle accidents
- Motor pedestrian collisions
- Epidemiology
  o 13-16% of pelvic ring fractures

Classification of Pelvic Ring Fractures
- Vertical shear pelvic fracture
- Lateral compression pelvic fracture
- Anterior compression pelvic fracture

Clinical Issues
Presentation
- Pelvic pain
- Pelvic instability

Natural History
- Overall mortality in pelvic ring fractures is approximately 6%
  o Pelvic hemorrhage 39%
  o Traumatic brain injury 31%
  o Multiple organ failure 30%
- Immediate complications
  o Pelvic hemorrhage in up to 75% of patients
  o Bladder injury
    - Extraperitoneal rupture due to pelvic fracture fragments
    - Intraperitoneal rupture less commonly associated with pelvic ring fracture
  o Urethral injury from shearing forces of the disrupted pelvic ring
  o Nerve injury
    - Sacral plexus
    - Sacral nerve roots
    - Sciatic nerve
- Early and late complications
  o Thromboembolic disease
  o Pain
  o Malunion
  o Osteoarthritis
  o Impotence

Treatment
- Immediate stabilization with external fixator devices to decrease hemorrhage
- Embolization for uncontrollable hemorrhage
- Open reduction and internal fixation
  o Open book fracture with more than 2.5 cm pubic symphysis diastasis
- Surgery may be indicated when there are concomitant genitourinary injuries

Prognosis
- Related to residual deformity after treatment

Selected References
1. Hunter JC et al: Pelvic and acetabular trauma. Radiol Clin North Am. 35:559-90, 1997
2. Tile M: Pelvic ring fractures: should they be fixed? J Bone Joint Surg Br. 70 :1-12, 1988
3. Young JW et al: Pelvic fractures: Value of plain radiography in early assessment and management. Radiology. 160:445-51, 1986

Acetabular Fracture

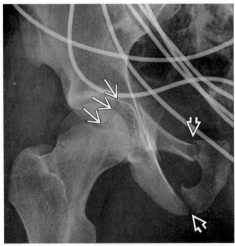

Acetabular Fracture. Coned down radiograph of the right hip shows a fracture (arrows) extending through the posterior wall of the acetabulum. Additional fractures of the superior and inferior pubic rami are noted (open arrows).

Key Facts
- Definition: Fracture of the anatomic components of acetabulum
- Classic imaging appearance: Discontinuity of the acetabular landmarks
- Other key facts: Often associated with posterior hip dislocation
- Classification
  - Posterior wall: One third of acetabular fractures
  - Transverse: Fracture is oriented from anterior to posterior
    - T-type: Transverse fracture with a vertical component
  - Columns: Fracture is in coronal plane through the roof of the acetabulum
    - Anterior
    - Posterior
    - Both columns: Accounts for up to 25% of all acetabular fractures

Imaging Findings
<u>General Features</u>
- Identification of the following landmarks
  - Iliopectineal line
  - Ilioischial line
  - Acetabular roof
  - Tear drop sign
  - Anterior acetabular lip
  - Posterior acetabular lip
  - Iliac wing
  - Obturator foramen
- Anatomy
  - Pelvis is referred to as an inverted Y: Ilium is the vertical limb, anterior and posterior columns are the respective columns and the acetabulum lies at their insertion

Acetabular Fracture

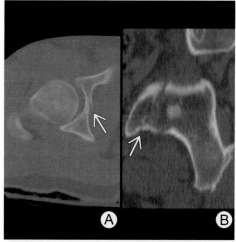

Acetabular Fracture. (A) Initial axial CT image of the right hip shows minimally displaced fracture of the medial wall (arrow). (B) Sagittal reformatted CT image in a different patient shows comminuted fracture of the acetabular roof (arrow).

- o Anterior column: Anterior aspect of the iliac wing, pelvic brim, superior pubic ramus, anterior wall of the acetabulum, and the teardrop
- o Posterior column: Posterior ilium, the posterior articular surface and posterior wall of the acetabulum, the ischium and most of the quadrilateral plate

Radiographic Findings
- AP pelvis: May show disruption of iliopectineal and ilioischial lines
- Pelvic obturator oblique
  - o Fractures of anterior column of the acetabulum and the posterior rim
  - o Discontinuity of the obturator foramen, which is seen in its largest dimension
- Pelvic iliac oblique
  - o Greater and lesser sciatic notches seen
  - o Any involvement of the posterior column of the acetabulum
  - o The anterior rim profiled
  - o The iliac wing seen in its largest dimension

CT Findings
- NECT
  - o Fractures of the quadrilateral surface
  - o Position and orientation of the intraarticular free fragments
  - o The orientation of the fracture line

MR Findings
- T1WI: Fracture appears as linear low signal
- STIR: Linear high signal
- Evaluation of ligamentous and also muscle injuries

Imaging Recommendations
- AP and Judet radiographs
  - o Initial evaluation method
  - o Identification of the presence of fracture

Acetabular Fracture

- CT with reformats
  - o Further detailed evaluation and preoperative planning
- 3D CT
  - o Good overall picture of acetabular fractures
- MRI maybe valuable for evaluation of occult fractures and also evaluation of soft tissue injury

Differential Diagnosis
Os Acetabuli Marginalis Superior
- Normal variant: Secondary ossification centers
- Most commonly in the superior aspect of the posterior acetabular lip either unilaterally or bilaterally
- Usually appear around 16 years of age and may persist throughout adult life

Pathology
General
- Etiology-Pathogenesis
  - o Caused by a force applied to the femur, translated to the acetabulum
  - o In young adults, due to high-energy injuries, primarily motor vehicle collisions
  - o Minority of patients are elderly, who may suffer relatively minor trauma causing acetabular fractures

Clinical Issues
Presentation
- Pain, limited range of motion, swelling and bruising
Natural History
- If undiagnosed or untreated: Sciatic nerve palsy, heterotopic bone formation, infection, thrombophlebitis, avascular necrosis of the femoral head, post traumatic arthritis
Treatment
- Non-operative treatment
  - o Non-displaced acetabular fractures
  - o Transverse fractures
  - o Minimally displaced two-column fractures
- Urgent surgery
  - o Acetabular fractures with anterior or posterior hip dislocations that cannot be reduced by closed methods
Prognosis
- Following a concise and well thought out algorithm, good result with minimal long-term complications

Selected References
1. Blumberg ML: Computed tomography and acetabular trauma. Comput. Tomog. 4:47, 1980
2. Lansinger O: Fractures of the acetabulum. A clinical, radiological and experimental study. Acta Orthop. Scand. 165:1, 1977
3. Judet R et al: Fractures of the acetabulum: Classification and surgical approaches for open reduction. J.Bone Joint Surg. 46:1615, 1964

PocketRadiologist®

ER-Trauma
Top 100 Diagnoses

LOWER EXTREMITY INJURY

Hip Dislocation

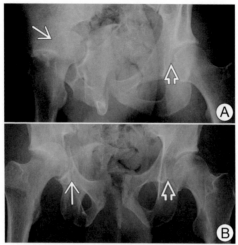

Hip Dislocation. (A) Oblique view of the pelvis demonstrates posterior dislocation of the femoral head (arrow). Note the contralateral normal side (open arrow). (B) AP pelvis on the same patient shows posterior pelvic rim fracture in posterior hip dislocation (arrow). Note the contralateral normal side (open arrow).

Key Facts
- Definition: Disruption of the joint relationship between the femoral head and the acetabulum
- Classic imaging appearance: Femoral head in a non anatomical location
- Classification
  - Posterior hip dislocation
  - Anterior hip dislocation
  - Central acetabular fracture-dislocation

Imaging Findings
General Features
- Best imaging clue
  - Posterior dislocation: Lateral and superior displacement of the femoral head
  - Anterior dislocation: Femoral head displaced into the obturator, pubic, or iliac area
  - Central dislocation: Femoral head protrudes into the pelvic cavity
- Anatomy
  - Femur is held in the acetabulum by five separate ligaments
  - Blood supply
    - Proximal femoral shaft and the femoral neck: Femoral artery
    - Femoral head: Poor blood supply from obturator artery

Radiographic Findings
- AP pelvis
  - Provides information about the type of dislocation
  - Fractures of the posterior rim of the acetabulum
- Lateral and oblique views of the hip
  - Fractures of the femoral head, neck, and acetabulum

Hip Dislocation

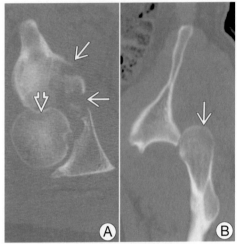

Hip dislocation. (A) Axial CT image through the pelvis shows posterior location of the right femoral head. Note the fractures of the acetabulum (arrows) and the femoral head (open arrow). (B) Sagittal reformatted CT image confirms posterior dislocation of the right hip (arrow).

CT Findings
- NECT
  - Delineating the extent and nature of hip fractures and dislocations
  - Evaluation of intrarticular fracture fragments
- CECT: Evaluation of vascular injury with CT angiogram

MR Findings
- T1WI: Low signal indicating effusion within the joint
- T2WI: High signal of the joint effusion, the injured ligaments and muscles

Imaging Recommendations
- Pre and post reduction radiographs for initial evaluation of abnormality
  - AP pelvis including both hips
  - AP and lateral of the affected hip
- MDCT: Detailed assessment of the fracture dislocation and preop planning
  - 1.25 mm axial images
    - Soft tissue and bone algorithms
  - Sagittal and coronal reformations
- MRI of the hip is impractical in the initial evaluation, however the best imaging modality in detecting
  - Fractures, in radiographically occult cases
  - Associated AVN of the femoral head
  - Nondisplaced stress fractures of the femoral neck
    - Coronal and axial T1W, coronal and axial FSE T2W F/S

Differential Diagnosis

Fractures of the Femur and also Fractures of the Acetabulum
- Femoral head is located
- May be associated with dislocation

Hip Dislocation

Pathology
<u>General</u>
- Etiology-Pathogenesis: High-speed, high-impact sports
  - Posterior hip dislocation
    - Flexed knee strikes dashboard with adducted legs
    - Fall with landing on the feet
  - Anterior hip dislocation
    - Posterior seat passenger with abducted legs and a valgus force
    - Direct blow to the posterior aspect of the hip
  - Central acetabular fracture-dislocation
    - Lateral force applied to the greater trochanter
- Epidemiology
  - Approximately 5% of all dislocations
    - Posterior hip dislocations in up to 90% of cases
  - Down's syndrome patients are predisposed to hip dislocations

Clinical Issues
<u>Presentation</u>
- Severe pain in the hip, upper leg, knee, lower leg, or even back pain
- Inability to walk or move the leg around the hip joint
- Posterior hip dislocations: Paresis/numbness in the sciatic nerve distribution
- Anterior hip dislocations
  - Paresis/numbness in the femoral nerve distribution
  - Injury to the femoral artery may cause pain, pallor, paresthesias
<u>Natural History</u>
- Avascular necrosis of the femoral head, high incidence of deep venous thrombosis, early osteoarthritis
<u>Treatment</u>
- Closed reduction within 6 hours of initial diagnosis
  - Subsequent traction and non weight-bearing immobilization
- Open reduction and internal fixation indicated in cases of
  - Irreducible dislocation
  - Persistent instability of the joint following reduction
  - Fracture of the femoral head or shaft
  - Neurovascular deficits that occur after closed reduction
<u>Prognosis</u>
- Overall, good to excellent results are obtained in up to 90% of patients

Selected References
1. Erb RE et al: Traumatic anterior dislocation of the hip: Spectrum of plain film and CT findings. A.J.R. 165:1215, 1995
2. Jacob JR et al: Traumatic dislocation and fracture dislocation of the hip. Clin. Orthop. 214:249, 1987
3. Reigstad A: Traumatic dislocation of the hip. J. Trauma. 20:603, 1980

Femoral Neck Fracture

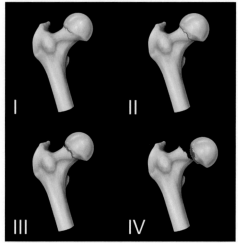

Garden classification of subcapital femoral fractures. (I) Incomplete with impaction of lateral cortex. (II) Complete with impaction. (III) Complete, partially displaced. Must have one fracture surface in apposition posteriorly and inferiorly. (IV) Complete, full displacement with no contact of fracture surfaces.

Key Facts
- Synonym(s): Transcervical fracture, subcapital fracture, midcervical fracture, basicervical fracture
- Definition: Fracture line traversing the femoral neck
- Classic imaging appearance
  - Fracture line crossing the femoral neck
  - May be displaced or non-displaced fracture line may be medial on the femoral neck at the junction of the femoral head, or anywhere along the neck toward the intertrochanteric ridge
- Femoral neck fracture classification
  - Midcervical or transcervical fracture
    - Rare
    - Fracture line separates femoral neck midway between head and intertrochanteric ridge
  - Basicervical fracture
    - Uncommon (insufficiency, stress, pathologic fracture)
    - Laterally placed fracture line separates femoral neck from intertrochanteric ridge
  - Subcapital fracture
    - Most common
    - Usually a short spiral fracture close to the epiphyseal scar
    - Separates femoral neck from head
    - May be impacted, displaced, complete or incomplete

Imaging Findings
General Features
- Best imaging clue: In most common form, the subcapital fracture shows a disruption in the medial cortex, creating a "spike" of bone
- Head may rotate into a valgus position (AP view) giving a "mushroom cap" appearance

Femoral Neck Fracture

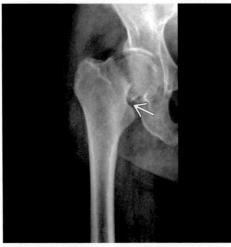

Subcapital fracture of the femoral neck. The fracture is complete and displaced (garden IV). The femoral head fragment fractures from the femoral neck, leaving a free edge "spike" of bone on the medial inferior aspect of the head fragment (arrow). A cortical defect is seen in this position on non-displaced fractures.

- Variable posterior rotation (true lateral view)

<u>CT Findings</u>
- Coronal and sagittal reformations are critical in making the diagnosis
- Minimally or non-displaced fractures may be misconstrued as hypertrophic osteoarthropathy or missed entirely on axial images
- Coronal reformations allow identification of impaction lines, medial head rotation and any comminuted segments

<u>MR Findings</u>
- T1WI May show a hypointense fracture line in marrow space
- T2WI Hyperintense marrow space edema around fracture site
  - Fat suppression increases sensitivity
    - T2WI with chemical fat saturation or STIR
- MRI/A attempts to identify vascular injury have not been helpful for predicting risk of avascular necrosis

<u>Other Modality Findings</u>
- Tc-99m bone scan reveals uptake in site of active repair: Useful for finding occult, non-displaced fractures

<u>Imaging Recommendations</u>
- Plain film is first evaluation: Should include AP, and true lateral or groin lateral
- CT with sagittal and coronal reformations may be obtained to classify difficult fractures
- MRI helpful in cases of subtle, minimally displaced incomplete fractures

Differential Diagnosis

<u>Midcervical Fracture, Basicervical Fracture</u>
- Fracture line is more distal than subcapital, further from femoral head
- Garden classification scheme does not apply

Femoral Neck Fracture

Pathology
- None relevant to this case

Clinical Issues
Presentation
- Ranges from hip pain to unable to bear weight with inward rotation of leg

Natural History
- Major determinant of healing is uninjured superior epiphyseal artery
- The more displaced the femoral head, more likely injured artery

Treatment
- Nondisplaced or incomplete fractures treated with non-weight bearing rest
- Displaced fractures must be reduced and fixed with nail

Prognosis
- Avascular necrosis occurs in 1 year on the average, and ranges from 8% in nondisplaced fracture to 30% with displaced femoral head
- Tc bone scan helpful in identifying blood flow and predicting risk of AVN
- Nonunion occurs in about 25%
- After pinning, 5-10% yearly incidence: After 5 years, can occur in 35% with united fractures

Selected References
1. Cuckler JM et al: An algorithm for the management of femoral neck fractures. Orthopedics. 17(9):789-92, 1994
2. Schwappach JR et al: Subcapital fractures of the femoral neck: prevalence and cause of radiographic appearance simulating pathologic fracture. AJR Am J Roentgenol. 162(3):651-4, 1994
3. Garden RS; Reduction and fixation of subcapital fractures of the femur. Orthop Clin North Am.; 5(4):683-712, 1974

Intertrochanteric Femur Fracture

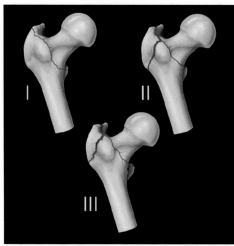

Three configurations of intertrochanteric fracture: I: Two-part fracture. II: Three-part fracture. Greater trochanter fragment shown here, but may have lesser trochanteric fragment. III: Four-part with neck/head, greater, lesser and proximal femur fragments.

Key Facts
- Definition: Proximal hip fracture in which the fracture line passes from the greater to lesser trochanter parallel to the intertrochanteric ridge
- Classic imaging appearance: Fracture plane oriented in the supra-lateral to infero-medial direction extending from the greater to lesser trochanters on frontal plain film
- RARELY incomplete
- About 50% are stable
- May have multiple fragments
  - ~ 25% are two fragment fractures
  - ~ 60% have three or more fragments
  - ~ 15% highly comminuted, might pass to subtrochanteric area
- In RARE cases, fracture line may be opposite expected – supra-medial to infero-lateral across intertrochanteric ridge
  - Typically occur low; start at lesser trochanter, pass laterally across intertrochanteric ridge into the subtrochanteric region
  - May not be evident on the AP view

Imaging Findings
General Features
- Fracture plane oriented in the supra-lateral to infero-medial direction extending from the greater to lesser trochanters
- Degree of separation of the fracture fragments is variable
- Classification system
  - Two-part fracture
    - 1: Femoral head and neck fragment
    - 2: Both trochanters and proximal femur
  - Three-part fracture
    - 1: Femoral head and neck fragment

Intertrochanteric Femur Fracture

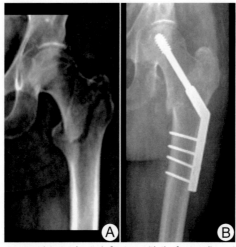

(A) Shows a two-part intertrochanteric fracture with the fracture line extending from the greater to lesser trochanters. (B) Shows the fracture after fixation with a dynamic compression screw. Note that the screw passes across the fracture line with the threads in the femoral head.

- 2: Trochanteric fragment: Greater trochanter fragment OR lesser trochanter fragment
- 3: Proximal femur and remaining attached trochanter
- o Four-part fracture
  - 1: Femoral head and neck fragment
  - 2: Greater trochanter fragment
  - 3: Lesser trochanter fragment
  - 4: Proximal femur fragment
- o Stability
  - May be stable (~ 50%): Two-part fractures; three-part fracture with free lesser trochanter
  - Consider all others unstable

CT Findings
- Fracture line follows intertrochanteric ridge of femur
- 2D axial and coronal reformatted views help define fracture lines and separated fragments
- 3D imaging may be helpful for planning placement of compression plate

Imaging Recommendations
- Plain film is typically sufficient to identify and classify fractures
- If needed, CT can define complex fracture planes
- MRI, T1WI, T2WI or STIR may help identify occult fracture lines

Differential Diagnosis

Subtrochanteric Fracture
- Fracture line distal to intertrochanteric ridge

Basi-Cervical Fracture
- Fracture line through femoral neck above intertrochanteric ridge

Intertrochanteric Femur Fracture

Pathology
- None relevant to this case

Clinical Issues
Presentation
- Predominantly in elderly
- Unable to bear weight
- Foot of affected hip rotated inward

Treatment
- If treated with traction (closed) – morbidity and mortality 5-10%
  - Elderly patient in traction susceptible to complications
- Open fixation
  - Jewett nail
    - Nail and compression plate fixed to lateral shaft cortex
  - Dynamic compression screw
    - Allows for settling the fragments on weight bearing
    - Screw backs out through sleeve as the fragments settle into each other

Prognosis
- Non-union and aseptic necrosis ~ 1%
- Good blood supply; vessels unlikely to be injured in this fracture

Selected References
1. Watson JT et al: Ipsilateral femoral neck and shaft fractures: Complications and their treatment. Clin Orthop. (399):78-86, 2002
2. Craig JG et al: Fractures of the greater trochanter: Intertrochanteric extension shown by MR imaging. Skeletal Radiol. 29(10):572-6, 2000
3. Yu JS: Hip and femur trauma. Semin Musculoskelet Radiol. 4(2):205-20, 2000

Femoral Shaft Fracture

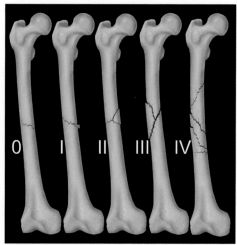

Winquist and Hansen classification. See text for details of the classification scheme. As fracture becomes more comminuted, less of the proximal and distal fragments remain in contact. With diminishing contact, the fracture is considered less stable. Stability decreases from type 0 (most stable) to IV (least stable).

Key Facts
- Definition: A fracture of the femur anywhere along the shaft from about 5 cm distal to the lesser trochanter (below the subtrochanteric region) and proximal to the distal femur at the point where it begins to flare into the supracondylar segment
- Classic imaging appearance: Most commonly occur in the middle third of the femoral shaft
- In children and adolescents, may rarely be incomplete
  - "Bowing fracture"
  - Bent, but no clear fracture fragments
  - Compare to contralateral extremity
  - Bone scan or MRI may be helpful
  - Asymmetrically thickened cortex when healed
- Violent forces needed to break the mid femoral shaft
  - Motor vehicle collision
  - Gunshot wound
  - Child abuse
  - Not common in the elderly, unless insufficiency due to co-existing disease
- Fracture line most commonly transverse or oblique
  - Minimal comminution at the margins
- Subtle incomplete fractures connected by a small bridge of intact bone MUST be identified
  - High complication rate in placing intramedullary rod
  - Femur tends to shatter along the bridging bone
- Due to the violent forces needed to break the femur, there is a high incidence of associated injury
  - Head, chest and abdominal visceral injury in about 25%
  - Ipsilateral bony injury of the lower extremity or pelvis in ~ 20%

Femoral Shaft Fracture

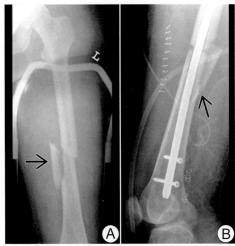

(A) Type III mid shaft femur fracture. Note large butterfly fragment (A, B arrow) with small (< 50%) contact between main fragments. (B) Lateral view of the same fracture after placement of intramedullary nail. Locking screws are seen distally crossing both the nail and the distal femoral metaphysis

Imaging Findings
<u>General Features</u>
- Can be classified by the method of Winquist and Hansen
  - Type 0
    - No comminution
  - Type I
    - Single free butterfly fragment
    - Butterfly fragment is tiny
    - Has no impact on fracture stability
  - Type II
    - Single free butterfly fragment
    - Larger than in type I
    - Maintains > 50% direct cortical contact between the main proximal and distal fragments
  - Type III
    - Single free butterfly fragment
    - Larger than in type I or II
    - < 50% direct connection remains between the main proximal and distal fragments
  - Type IV
    - Multiple comminuted segments
    - Segmental fracture fragments separate the main proximal and distal femur fragments
    - No direct contact between the main proximal and distal fragments
- Stability decreases with for advanced fracture type
- Fractures may be open or closed
  - Segmental fragments my be displaced outside the patient in open fractures

Femoral Shaft Fracture

CT Findings
- CT is not indicated in identifying and classifying femoral shaft fractures
- Multi-detector CT arteriogram can be used to identify arterial dissection and laceration with extravasation
  - Vascular injury UNCOMMON in proximal and mid shaft fractures
  - More common in distal shaft injury, in area of adductor canal

MR Findings
- May be indicated to identify soft tissue injury
  - Muscle hematoma or tear
  - Nerve or vessel injury
- T1WI Iso to slightly hyperintense signal causing mass effect in muscle
- T2WI Hyperintense signal in hematoma causes mass effect and displacement of local hypointense muscle
  - Hyperintensity in muscle tissue may indicate strain
- MRA In open or severely angulated fractures, look for arterial dissection or pseudoaneurysm

Imaging Recommendations
- AP and lateral views are typically sufficient to identify and classify the femoral fracture
  - If questions about incomplete fracture, oblique views may be performed to confirm continuity of bone
- CTA or MRA for question of vascular injury
- MRI > CT for soft tissue injury

Differential Diagnosis
- None relevant to this case

Pathology
- None relevant to this case

Clinical Issues

Presentation
- Deformity, discoloration, pain and swelling in the thigh following trauma

Treatment
- Closed reduction - traction
  - Pins placed across distal femur or proximal tibia
- Open reduction
  - Children - traction and hip spica cast
    - Often allow ~ 1 cm overlap of fragments
    - Allows for overgrowth during healing
    - Avoids limb length discrepancy
  - Adults - intramedullary rod/nail
    - Driven through the marrow cavity across fracture
    - May be "locked" into place proximally and distally
    - Screws traverse bone, pass through nail
    - Prevents shortening and rotation on settling

Selected References
1. Winquist RA et al: Closed intramedullary nailing of femoral fractures. A report of five hundred and twenty cases - 1984. J Bone Joint Surg Am. 83-A(12):1912, 2001
2. Bouchard et al: Outcome of femoral shaft fractures in the elderly. Clin Orthop. (332):105-9, 1996
3. Winquist RA et al: Comminuted fractures of the femoral shaft treated by intramedullary nailing. Orthop Clin North Am. 11:633-48, 1980

Patellar Fracture

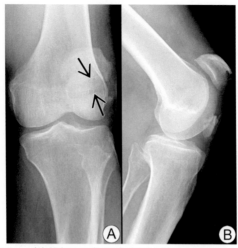

Patellar Fracture. (A) AP knee radiograph shows a transverse fracture through the distal third of the patella (arrows). (B) Lateral knee radiograph shows a widely distracted and comminuted patella fracture.

Key Facts
- Synonym: Knee cap fracture
- Definition: Traumatic disruption of the patella
- Classic imaging appearance
  - Transversely oriented lucent fracture line across middle or distal third of patella

Imaging Findings
General Features
- 60% transversely oriented
  - Usually undisplaced
- 25% are comminuted
  - More often displaced
- 15% vertically oriented
  - Usually undisplaced and difficult to visualize on standard AP and lateral radiographs

Radiography Findings
- Fracture may be obscured on the AP view due to overlying femur
- Lateral views more clearly demonstrate fracture
  - Better able to asses separation and comminution

CT Findings
- Primarily used for radiographically occult fractures
  - Coronal and sagittal reformations helpful in defining position of fracture fragments

MR Findings
- Also useful in radiographically occult fractures
- Useful in evaluating for soft tissue injury
  - Chondral defects
  - Retinacular attachments
  - Quadriceps and patellar tendon injury

Patellar Fracture

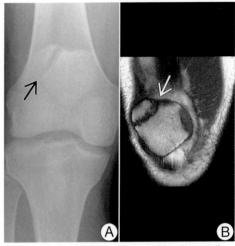

Bipartite patella. (A) AP radiograph shows a bipartite patella. The defect characteristically extends through the superior-lateral portion of patella (arrow). Note the parallel sclerotic margins. (B) Coronal FSE T1MR image in another patient also shows a bipartite patella (arrow).

- o Loose bodies
- Helpful in differentiating patellar fracture from the lengthy differential diagnosis

<u>Imaging Recommendations</u>
- Standard AP and lateral views usually adequate for transverse and comminuted fractures
- Patella (sunrise, sunset) view helpful in identifying vertical fractures
- Radiographs of contralateral knee may confirm bipartite patella
  - o Bipartite patella is rarely unilateral
- Nuclear medicine
  - o Bone scintigraphy
    - May be useful as a complementary modality in evaluating stress fractures and bipartite patella

Differential Diagnosis
<u>Bipartite Patella</u>
- Important to distinguish from patellar fracture
- Discrete secondary patella ossification center
- Sclerotic margins
  - o Smoothly parallel
  - o Superior lateral margin of patella
- M:F = 9:1
- 2% of population

<u>Patellar Dislocation</u>
- No fracture on imaging studies
- AP film shows lateral displacement of patella
- MRI shows characteristic pattern of injury in patellar dislocation
  - o Contusion and cartilage defect of the medial patellar facet
  - o Contusion of lateral femoral condyle

Patellar Fracture

- o Injury to the medial retinaculum

<u>Patellar or Quadriceps Tendon Rupture</u>
- No fracture on imaging studies
- Patella elevated with patella tendon rupture
- Patella displaced inferiorly with quadriceps tendon rupture
- Both tendon ruptures easily visualized on MRI

<u>Sinding-Larsen-Johansson Syndrome</u>
- Osteochondrosis of the distal pole at origin of patellar tendon
  - o Multiple ossific fragments at origin of patellar tendon

Pathology
- Etiology-Pathogenesis
  - o Result from direct trauma to patella
  - o Also occurs with forceful contraction of the quadriceps muscle when the knee is flexed
- Epidemiology
  - o 1% of all skeletal injuries in both adults and children

Clinical Issues
<u>Presentation</u>
- Patellar pain with a history of direct or indirect injury
- Knee joint effusion

<u>Natural History</u>
- Complications
  - o Nonunion
  - o Posttraumatic osteoarthritis
  - o Avascular necrosis
  - o Quadriceps weakness

<u>Treatment</u>
- Transverse fracture
  - o Open reduction and fixation
- Comminuted fracture
  - o May require total patellectomy if severely comminuted
- Vertical fracture
  - o May only require casting if fracture minimally displaced (2-3 mm)

<u>Prognosis</u>
- Posttraumatic osteoarthritis more common in previously injured knees

Selected References
1. Carpenter JE et al: Biomechanical evaluation of current patella fracture fixation techniques. J Orthop Trauma. 15:351-6, 1997
2. Yu JS et al: MR imaging of injuries of the extensor mechanism of the knee. Radiographics. 14:541-51, 1994
3. Ray JM et al: Incidence, mechanism of injury, and treatment of fractures of the patella in children. J Trauma. 32:464-7, 1992

Knee Dislocation

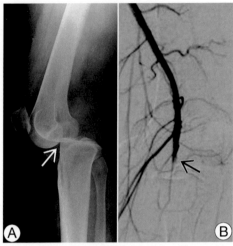

Posterior dislocation of knee: Tibia is displaced posterior with respect to distal femur. Note impact of femur on anterior tibial plateau (A, arrow). Post reduction angiogram of same patient shows tapering and then truncation of contrast in this traumatic dissection of popliteal artery (B, arrow).

Key Facts

- Definition: Complete disruption of stabilizing ligaments of tibiofemoral joint with displacement of tibia with respect to femur
- Classic imaging appearance anteroposterior and/or lateromedial misalignment of tibia with respect to femur on AP and lateral plain films
- True dislocation of tibiofemoral joint is rare
- Dislocation is named for position of tibia with respect to femur (i.e. anterior dislocation has tibia in front of femur)
  - Anterior dislocation most common type (~30%)
    - Typically hyperextension mechanism
    - Ligament injury
    - Posterior joint capsule torn
    - Anterior cruciate ligament (ACL) torn
    - Posterior cruciate ligament (PCL) variable
    - Collateral ligaments often spared
  - Posterior dislocation less common (~25%)
    - Usually direct impact mechanism, ACL and PCL torn, extensor mechanism injured
  - Transverse dislocation least common
    - Lateral (10%) - Medial (5%), posterolateral rotatory (5%), vessels (popliteal artery and vein) injury in ~30% of knee dislocations
  - Incidence of vessel injury increases directly with impact velocity
  - Posterior dislocation directly impacts vessels
    - Results in shearing force that transects artery
  - Anterior dislocation likely to stretch and dissect artery

Knee Dislocation

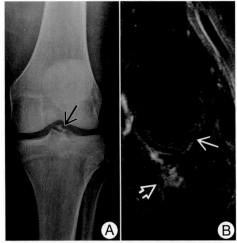

Reduced posterior dislocation: Avulsion fracture of anterior tibial eminence shown on AP radiograph (A, arrow) T2WI with fat suppression in same knee shows free distal end of torn ACL (B, arrow). Anterior tibial plateau hyperintensity from femoral impact injury can also be seen (open arrow).

- Artery tethered at adductor hiatus and arch of soleus
- Peroneal nerve injury in ~20% of all knee dislocations

Imaging Findings
General Features
- Best imaging clue: Misaligned tibia and femur on AP and lateral views
- Subtle observations may indicate previous complete dislocation with spontaneous reduction
  - Unstable knee on physical examination
  - Widening of tibiofemoral joint
    - May be symmetric or asymmetric
  - Avulsion fracture of the anterior eminence of the tibia
    - ACL torn in all dislocation types
  - True lateral profile of femur and rotated appearance of tibia

CT Findings
- NECT with sagittal, coronal & 3D reformation helpful if fracture dislocation
- Usually not necessary as dislocation typically without fracture
  - May be helpful in identifying subtle tibial plateau fractures
    - Injury to ACL may result in anterior tibial eminence

MR Findings
- T1WI delineates anatomic detail and hypointense marrow bruise
  - Blood products in joint capsule iso to hyperintense
- T2WI with fat suppression or STIR sequence
  - Marrow space hyperintensity in bruising or subchondral injury
  - Hyperintense signal and fibrous disruption in ligament or tendon injury
  - Altered cartilaginous architecture and hyperintensity
- Proton density sequence provides excellent contrast between fat, muscle and fibrous tendons and ligaments

- o Arterial flow voids pronounced in plane orthogonal to direction of flow
- Arteriography
  - o MRA, CTA or conventional arteriogram to define popliteal artery
    - Gadolinium MRA more sensitive than 2D time of flight
- Low flow velocity or blood product "shine through" on 2D sequence may confuse appearance
- Dynamic Gd enhanced MRA provides contrast proportional to contrast blood concentration, giving more accurate depiction of lumen

Imaging Recommendations
- Imaging should begin with plain film evaluation in the AP, lateral and if possible at least one, but preferably both oblique projections
- Although rare, fracture dislocations may occur
- In these cases, NECT with sagittal, coronal & 3D reformations helpful
- If vascular injury is suspected, angiography using CTA, MRA or conventional arteriographic runoff should be performed
- MRI can be performed to evaluate ligament and tendon injury prior to surgical reduction and stabilization

Differential Diagnosis
Patellar Dislocation
- Although knee joint itself remains intact, patient describes a "pop" and a feeling of motion in knee at time of stress
- Much more common than true knee dislocation
- Happens on "cutting" or rapid change in direction while running
  - o Tibia flexed, abducted and in valgus position, femur internally rotated, quadriceps contracts, pulling patella laterally
- Plain film shows normal knee joint alignment and architecture
- Lateral patellar dislocation most common

Pathology
- None relevant to this case

Clinical Issues
Presentation
- Pain, instability and deformity in knee joint after violent mechanism
- If distal pulses are present, likelihood of arterial injury is low
  - o Pulse may still be present in significant vascular injury

Treatment & Prognosis
- Pain and swelling control
- Initial reduction and immobilization
- Imaging to define ligamentous injury
  - o Delay imaging 7-10 days to allow for swelling to decrease
- Repair joint alignment and stability by open reduction and ligament repair
- If lower extremity vessel injury is present and repair of vessel is delayed > 8 hours, ~80% amputation rate
- If vessel injury is repaired within 8 hours, ~80% limb salvage rate

Selected References
1. Martinez D et al: Popliteal artery injury associated with knee dislocations. Am Surg 67(2): 165-7, 2001
2. Almekinders LC: Outcomes of the operatively treated knee dislocation. Clin Sports Med. 19(3): 503-18, 2000
3. Brautigan B et al: The epidemiology of knee dislocations. Clin Sports Med 19(3): 387-97, 2000

Tibial Plateau Fracture

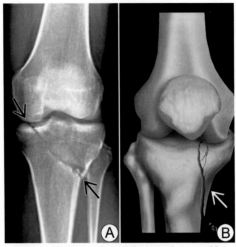

Tibial plateau fracture. (A) AP view through the knee shows an oblique line through the medial tibial plateau, extending laterally into the tibial neck (arrows). (B) Drawing of the knee of another case shows the relations of the split fracture of the medial tibial plateau with adjacent structures (arrow).

Key Facts
- Synonyms: Bumper fracture; fender fracture; broken knee
- Definition: Disruption of the tibial condyles
- Classic imaging appearance
  - Elderly: Usually compression fracture with decreased height of tibial plateau and subjacent sclerotic line
  - Young adults: Usually splitting fracture through the tibial plateau with a lucent line
- Associated with
  - Injuries to the cruciate and collateral ligaments
  - Fracture of the fibular head
- Classification: (Schatzker classification)
  - Type I: Pure cleavage fractue of the lateral plateau
  - Type II: Cleavage and compression fractures of the lateral plateau
  - Type III: Pure compression fracture of the lateral plateau
  - Type IV: Medial plateau fracture with a split (splinter fragment) or depressed comminution
  - Type V: Bicondylar fracture
  - Type VI: Combined transverse fracture of the tibial neck with oblique fracture of the lateral tibial plateau

Imaging Findings
General Features
- Best imaging clue
  - Younger patients: Pattern of fracture is splitting
  - Older patients: Pattern of fracture is depression
- Anatomy
  - Tibia is composed of the medial and lateral tibial plateaus, as well as the intercondylar eminence

Tibial Plateau Fracture

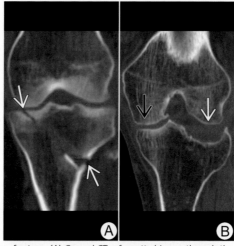

Tibial plateau fracture. (A) Coronal CT reformatted image through the knee shows fracture of the medial plateau in a young patient (arrows). (B) Coronal CT reformatted image through the knee in a different older patient shows fracture of the lateral tibial plateau (white arrow), normal medial tibial plateau (black arrow).

- Medial plateau of the tibia is stronger than the lateral plateau
  - Ligaments
    - Anterior and posterior cruciate ligaments
    - Lateral and medial collateral ligaments

Radiography Findings
- AP radiograph of the knee
  - Fracture lucency in split fractures
  - Sclerotic line in depressed fractures with decreased height
- Cross-table lateral radiograph: The most important view to detect occult fractures
  - Lipohemarthrosis is indicative of occult fractures

CT Findings
- Assessment of the depression of the tibial plateau
- Assessment of the degree of splitting of the fractured fragments

MR Findings
- T1WI: Anatomic information
  - Splitt fractures: Low signal line
  - Depression fractures: Low signal bone marrow edema
- STIR: Rapidly performed and very sensitive
  - Absence of high signal excludes a fracture

Angiography Findings
- Arteriography: Indicated if popliteal artery injury is suspected

Imaging Recommendations
- Trauma setting: Cross-table lateral and anteroposterior (AP) views of the knee
- Preferred examination: AP, cross-table lateral, patellar (sunrise), oblique views
- MDCT
  - Slice thickness should be minimized (1.25 mm is ideal)

Tibial Plateau Fracture

- o Bone and soft tissue windows
- o Coronal and sagittal reformations
- MRI
  - o Trauma screening (fast MRI)
    - Coronal TI
    - Coronal STIR
  - o MR arthrography: Preferred method for evaluation of
    - Ligaments, menisci, intraarticular relations, intraarticular fracture fragments
    - T1 Fat saturated gadolinium enhanced sequences (arthrography) in coronal, sagittal and axial planes

Differential Diagnosis
Insufficiency Fractures of the Tibial Plateau
- Fracture of the osteoporotic bone with a physiologic force
- More common in older females as oppose to traumatic tibial plateau fractures which occur in young males
- More commonly involves the medial tibial plateau
- Sclerotic fracture line as oppose to lucent fracture line

Pathology
General
- Etiology-Pathogenesis
  - o Axial loading, such as from a fall (most common mechanism)
  - o Impact with automobile bumpers
  - o From laterally directed forces
  - o From a twisting injury
- Epidemiology
  - o Approximately 1% of all fractures involve the tibial plateau
  - o Fractures of the lateral tibial plateau are much more common

Clinical Issues
Presentation
- Knee effusion, pain, and joint stiffness
Natural History
- Early osteoarthritis, instability, articular discongruities, cartilage damage
Treatment
- Minimally displaced or depressed fractures
  - o Closed treatment and early mobilization
- Displaced or depressed fractures
  - o 4-5 mm of articular depression and 3-4 mm of diasthesis
  - o Open reduction and internal fixation
Prognosis
- Patients heal in most cases without complaints of instability

Selected References
1. Barrow BA et al: Tibial plateau fractures: evaluation with MR imaging. Radiographics. 14(3): 553-9, 1994
2. Anglen JO et al: Tibial plateau fractures. Orthopedics. 11:1527, 1988
3. Rafii M et al: Computed tomography of tibial plateau fractures. AJR. 142:1181, 1984

Tibia – Fibula Shaft Fractures

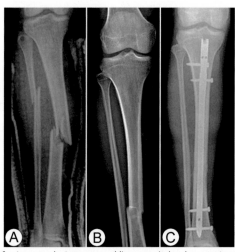

Tibial shaft fractures can be transverse, oblique or spiral and are most common in the middle and distal thirds of the shaft. Tibial fractures can occur with (A) or without (B) a fibula fracture. Open reduction with locking intramedullary nail placement (C) provides the greatest likelihood of good fracture healing.

Key Facts

- May be caused by direct or indirect forces
  - Direct forces typically present as transverse or comminuted fracture
  - Indirect forces typically present as spiral or oblique fracture
  - Repetitive loading such as in runners or other athletes may have focal failure of the cortex in compression = stress fracture
- Fractures more common in the middle and distal thirds of the shaft
- Tibial fractures are often accompanied by fibular fractures
  - Commonly occur at the same level
  - Frequently, fibula fracture will be more proximal to tibia fracture
    - Especially if caused by an indirect rotational force
    - Unstable because interosseous membrane often torn
  - In children, tibia often fractures WITHOUT fibula fracture
    - Fibula "bow fracture" may be present but subtle
    - Fibula appears bent, but no fracture line seen
- Fractures of the tibia may be accompanied by compartment syndrome
  - Three lower leg compartments: Anterior, posterior and lateral
  - Anterior compartment syndrome most common and worrisome
    - Pain, pallor, variable anterior tibial artery pulse, peroneal nerve palsy (weak dorsiflexion, sensory deficit)
    - Compartment bounded by tibia, fibula, interosseous membrane, deep fascia of the leg, tibiofibular diarthrosis and extensor retinaculum
    - Compartment contains tibialis anterior, extensor hallicus longus and extensor digitorum muscles, peroneal nerve and anterior tibial artery
    - Hemorrhage increases intra-compartment pressure
- Diminished arterial flow with tissue ischemia

Tibia – Fibula Shaft Fractures

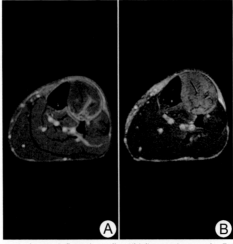

Compartment syndrome: Inflamed, swollen tibialis anterior muscle. Fat suppressed T1WI (A) shows central linear and peripheral enhancement in the enlarged muscle. T2WI (B) shows the homogeneously hyperintense muscle contained between the tibia, fibula, and interosseous membrane bounded anteriorly by leg fascia.

- Results in tissue edema and more pressure
- Eventually can lead to tissue necrosis

Imaging Findings
General Features
- Best imaging clue: Linear fracture line seen on plain film in longitudinal, transverse, oblique or spiral orientation
  - May be complete, incomplete, segmental or comminuted
- Spiral tibial fractures most common at junction of middle and distal third
  - Accompanying fibula fractures often just distal to fibular head

CT Findings
- In unusual cases where fracture fragments cannot be clearly delineated on plain film, nonenhanced CT with sagittal, coronal and 3D reformations may be helpful in preoperative planning
- CTA may be of use in cases where vascular injury is suspect
  - Arterial dissection or rupture with extravasation may be seen

MR Findings
- Chronically ischemic, atrophic muscle appears shrunken, T1 hyperintense, and T2 hypointense
- Hemorrhage may appear iso to slightly hyperintense to muscle on T1 and hyperintense and often heterogeneous on T2WI
- Edematous tissue appears expanded with diffusely hypointense signal on T1 and correspondingly hyperintense signal on T2WI
- MRA may be performed to evaluate the vasculature of the lower limb

Nuclear medicine
- In occult incomplete or stress fractures, bone scan makes the diagnosis by indicating the site of repair (hot spot)

Imaging Recommendations
- Plain film AP and lateral usually sufficient

Tibia – Fibula Shaft Fractures

- Oblique projection helpful in complex segmented or comminuted fractures
- CT generally not necessary, but may be occasionally helpful preoperatively in determining position of complex fracture fragments
- MRI to evaluate soft tissues for muscle or tendon injury
  - May be performed in chronic injury to evaluate for changes due to compartment syndrome

Pathology
- None relevant to this case

Differential Diagnosis
- None relevant to this case

Clinical Issues
Presentation
- Pain and deformation after direct impact trauma or rotational force
- Plain film should include ALL of lower leg from knee to ankle
  - Fractures may involve tibia, fibula or some combination
  - Fractures may be a multiple and at different levels
  - The degree of rotation of the fragments must be assessed both pre- and post reduction
- Compartment syndrome may require fasciotomy
Treatment
- Closed reduction is possible, but may have higher incidence of non or delayed union if incomplete apposition of fragments
- Open reduction and fixation reduces incidence of non or delayed union
  - Especially in spiral or complex segmental fractures
  - Fixation with locking intramedullary nail reduces likelihood of loading or rotation causing migration or misaligned fragments
Prognosis
- Healing is dependent on degree of comminution, displacement of fragments, open or closed injury and post op complications (i.e. infection)
  - Spiral tibial shaft fractures have high incidence of re-fracture and delayed union if not reduced completely
  - Open reduction with intramedullary nail reduces complications
- Tibial shaft fractures typically heal in ~16 weeks.
  - Consider delayed union if fracture line still seen at 20-22 weeks
  - Nonunion if still without callus or bridging at 6 months
    - Look for clear line with smooth, sclerotic borders
  - Distal third fractures more susceptible to non or delayed union
- Re-fracture is possible, especially in active patients (i.e. athletes)
  - May occur at old fracture line
  - May occur at gap site from a missing comminuted segment
  - May occur at screw hole from fixation device after removal

Selected References
1. French B et al: High-energy tibial shaft fractures. Orthop Clin North Am. 33(1): 211-30, ix, 2002
2. Karladani AH et al: The influence of fracture etiology and type on fracture healing: a review of 104 consecutive tibial shaft fractures. Arch Orthop Trauma Surg. 121(6): 325-8, 2001
3. Triffitt PD et al: Compartment pressures after closed tibial shaft fracture. Their relation to functional outcome. J Bone Joint Surg Br. 74(2): 195-8, 1992

Ankle Fractures - Tibia

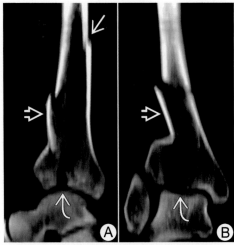

(A) Sagittal and (B) coronal CT reformations of a Pylon fracture demonstrate the shattered appearance of the distal tibia. The plafond is vertically disrupted in both planes (curved arrows). The anterolateral cortex is buckled (open arrows), and an oblique fracture is seen in the more proximal metaphysis (arrow).

Key Facts
<u>Common Ankle Fractures Involving the Tibia</u>
- Pylon (Pilon) fracture
  - Split or comminuted fracture of distal tibial plafond
  - Typically involves the anterior lip of the tibia
  - Axial loading fracture of the tibia
    - Jump from height or motor vehicle accident
    - Talus is driven up through the plafond
- Isolated posterior lip (Malleolus) fracture
  - Could occur by hyper plantar flexion mechanism
  - Exclude Weber B and Maisonneuve mechanisms
    - Supination external rotation but only if posterior lip of the tibia fractures just after tear of anteroinferior tibiofibular ligament with no oblique fibula fracture
    - Exclude proximal fibula fracture, medial malleolar fracture and disrupted syndesmosis
- Tillaux fracture
  - Foot external rotation mechanism
  - Avulsion fracture of the anterior tubercle of the tibia
    - Tension in the anterior tibiofibular ligament
  - If avulsion fracture of the fibula at attachment of the anterior tibiofibular ligament instead of anterior tibial tubercle, then called Wagstaff-Lefort fracture (rare)
- Tri-plane fracture
  - Children and young adults before closure of the growth plate
  - Plantar flexion with external rotation mechanism
  - Three fracture planes
    - Transverse fracture of the epiphyseal plate
    - Sagittal fracture of the epiphysis
    - Coronal distal metaphyseal fracture

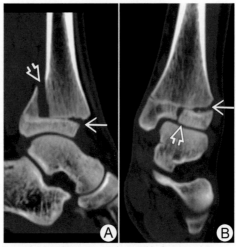

CT reformations of a two fragment tri-plane ankle fracture: A transverse fracture through the growth plate is seen on both views (A, B arrow). A coronal fracture is appreciated on the sagittal view (A, open arrow), while a sagittal fracture through the epiphysis is seen on the coronal view (B, open arrow).

- o Two types: Two fragment and three fragment
  - ▪ Two fragment variant more common
  - ▪ Occur after the epiphysis begins to unite
- Medial malleolar fractures may also be part of fibular fracture mechanisms

Imaging Findings

General Features
- Pylon: Disrupted plafond with variable widening and comminution
- Posterior malleolus: Best seen on lateral projection
- Tillaux: May be difficult to see on plain film - need CT
- Tri-plane: Misalignment on all projections centered on growth plate

CT Findings
- CT with coronal and sagittal reformation critical for defining fracture fragments as above for both classification and treatment planning

MR Findings
- T1 imaging not very helpful
- Hyperintense T2W signal in the marrow space may help identify bone bruising or fractures
- Proton density images provides excellent contrast to noise characteristics for following tendon course
- Heterogeneous signal in the usually dark tendons on T2 or PD images indicate tendon tear
  - o If separated edges can be seen, full thickness tear
  - o If increased signal with intact tendon margins, partial thickness
- Fat suppressed images aid in separating hyperintense T2 FSE or STIR signal indicating edema or hemorrhage from surrounding fat

Imaging Recommendations
- Plain films should be the initial modality for evaluating the ankle
  - o AP, lateral and mortise oblique views

- In complex or unstable injuries, CT with sagittal and coronal reformations provide needed detail to plan surgical fixation
- 3D reformations provide a global detail of fragment relationship helpful for planning reduction and fixation
- MRI helpful if tendon injury or entrapment is suspected

Differential Diagnosis
- None relevant to this case

Pathology
- None relevant to this case

Clinical Issues
Presentation
- Pain and deformity after ankle injury involving external rotation
- Instability and pain preclude weight bearing
Treatment
- Exact anatomic fracture reduction is key in all fractures
  - Most tri-plane fractures can be treated with closed reduction
    - If fracture crosses the growth plate with epiphysis and metaphysis fragments, open reduction may be needed
- Posterior malleolus fracture involving > 25-30% of the articulating surface likely require open reduction and internal fixation
- Complex comminuted (Pylon) fractures require open reduction fixation

Selected References
1. Borrelli J Jr et al: Pilon fractures: assessment and treatment. Orthop Clin North Am. 33(1):231-45, x, 2002
2. Karrholm J: The triplane fracture: four years of follow-up of 21 cases and review of the literature. J Pediatr Orthop B. 6(2):91-102, 1997
3. Solomon MA, et al: CT scanning of the foot and ankle: Clinical applications and review of the literature. AJR Am J Roentgenol. 146(6):1204-14, 1986

Ankle Fractures - Fibula

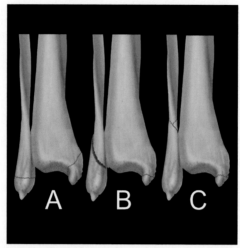

The Weber-Danis classification for ankle fractures: Fractures are classified by position of the fibular fracture line with respect to the mortise. Weber A shows a horizontal line below the mortise. Weber B has an oblique or spiral fracture beginning at the mortise. Weber C fractures begin above the mortise.

Key Facts
- Definition: The distal fibula forms the lateral malleolus of the ankle: Fractures of the distal fibula may contribute to instability of the ankle
- Classic imaging appearance: Fracture lucency with variably displaced distal fibular fragment
- Lauge-Hansen classification useful, but detailed and cumbersome
- Weber-Danis classification simple and useful in predicting mechanism and stability
- Classify injury by position of fracture on lateral malleolus with respect to the horizontal joint space
  - Weber A
    - Stable fracture
    - Supination-Adduction mechanism
    - Transverse fibular fracture below the level of the plafond
    - Talofibular and calcaneofibular ligaments may be injured
    - If there is an accompanying medial malleolus fracture, it is oblique
    - Deltoid ligament and tibio-fibular syndesmosis intact
  - Weber B
    - May be stable or unstable depending on ligamentous involvement
    - Supination-external rotation mechanism
    - Fibular fracture begins at the level of the plafond
    - Extends laterally in transverse or oblique direction
    - Oblique fracture best seen on lateral projection and may be missed altogether on frontal view
    - May also have fracture of the posterior malleolus
    - May have transverse medial malleolar fracture or tear of deltoid tendon

Ankle Fractures - Fibula

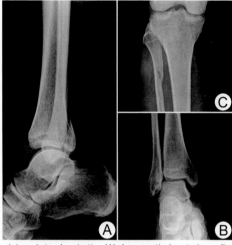

Maisonneuve injury: Lateral projection (A) shows vertical posterior malleolus fracture. Frontal projection (B) shows subtle widening of medial clear space of the ankle joint and tibio-fibular syndesmosis (better on oblique view). (C) Proximal fibular fracture (Maisonneuve fracture) is seen on inspection of the upper leg.

- o Weber C
  - ▪ Disruption of the tibiofibular syndesmosis common in fractures with this class of mechanism
  - ▪ More susceptible to transverse medial malleolar fracture or tear of deltoid tendon than Weber B
  - ▪ Ankle joint may be deranged: Look for widening of the medial or lateral clear space of the ankle (> 4 mm)
  - ▪ May also have posterior malleolus fracture
  - ▪ Unstable class of ankle fractures
  - ▪ Pronation-abduction mechanism (Weber C1): Fibula fracture just above the level of the plafond
  - ▪ Pronation-external rotation mechanism (Weber C2): Fibula fracture more proximal (up to 8 cm)
  - ▪ Maisonneuve injury (Weber C3): Disruption of tibiofibular syndesmosis and tear of interosseous membrane; Accompanied by proximal fibula shaft fracture, called "Maisonneuve fracture"; need film of the proximal fibula when this fracture is suspected
- • Dupytren's fracture is an eponym for
  - o Fracture of the fibula up to 10 cm proximal to the tibiofibular syndesmosis
  - o Tear of syndesmotic and interosseous ligaments
  - o Lateral displacement of the talus
  - o May have fracture of posterior malleolus

Imaging Findings
<u>General Features</u>
- • Best imaging clue: Fracture of the distal fibula
  - o Check position of fracture line with respect to ankle mortise

Ankle Fractures - Fibula

- Factors potentially affecting stability
  - Check tibiofibular syndesmosis for widening
    - Abnormal if > 5 mm in any projection
  - Displaced fractures of medial and posterior malleoli
    - May hint at disruption of syndesmosis or deltoid ligament, contributing to instability

CT Findings
- In general, CT is not needed for simple post-traumatic ankle injury involving the fibula

Imaging Recommendations
- Minimum 3 view plain film series to evaluate ankle
  - AP, Lateral and internal oblique (mortise) views
- AP supination or pronation stress views may be helpful if joint normal but suspected instability

Differential Diagnosis
Ankle Sprain
- Injury of the tibiofibular, talofibular or calcaneofibular ligaments, without fracture

Pathology
- None relevant to this case

Clinical Issues
Presentation
- Pain and swelling after "twisting ankle"

Treatment
- For stable fractures, closed anatomic reduction of the fracture with cast immobilization for 6-12 weeks
- For unstable fractures, open reduction and fixation
  - A variety of screw and plate combinations may be used
  - Fracture dislocation may be complicated by displacement or entrapment of tibialis posterior tendon

Selected References
1. Boutis K et al: Sensitivity of a clinical examination to predict need for radiography in children with ankle injuries: a prospective study. Lancet. 358(9299): 2118-21, 2001
2. Pinzur MS et al: Pitfalls in the treatment of fractures of the ankle and talus. Clin Orthop. (391): 17-25, 2001
3. Mulligan ME: Ankle fracture classifications clarified. Journal Abbrev. Radiology 5: 127-136, 1998

Tarsal Fractures

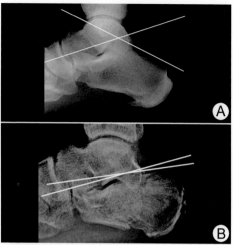

(A) Normal calcaneus has normal height and configuration. Boehler's angle is greater than 28°. (B) The tongue type calcaneal fracture shows fracture lines in the posterior tubercle and posterior facet with diminished height. When Boehler's angle is drawn, it is reduced to less than 28°.

Key Facts

- Injuries to the hindfoot (Talus and calcaneus) are more common than the midfoot (Navicula, Cuboid and Cuneiforms)
  - ○ Calcaneus is most common injury followed by talus
- Calcaneal fractures
  - ○ Boehler's Angle
    - ▪ Indicator of compromised calcaneal structural integrity
    - ▪ Measured on lateral view
    - ▪ First line between posterior superior margin of posterior calcaneal facet and anterior-superior tip of anterior process
    - ▪ Second line between the posterior superior margin of the posterior tubercle and the posterior superior margin of the posterior facet
    - ▪ Angle should not be less than 28 degrees
  - ○ Commonly compression type fractures
    - ▪ Result from excessive loading of the calcaneus
    - ▪ Fall from height landing on feet
    - ▪ About 75% involve the subtalar joint
    - ▪ Often comminuted
    - ▪ Two types: Tongue, centrolateral depression
- Talus fractures
  - ○ Most commonly talar neck fractures
  - ○ Talus can be dislocated with or without fracture
  - ○ Hawkins classification of talus fractures
    - ▪ Helps predict osteonecrosis of the talar dome
    - ▪ Vessels enter talar neck on its undersurface
    - ▪ Type I – Non-displaced fracture of the talar neck
    - ▪ Osteonecrosis approximately 10%
    - ▪ Type II – Mildly displaced neck fx and dislocated subtalar joint
    - ▪ Osteonecrosis approaches 40%

Tarsal Fractures

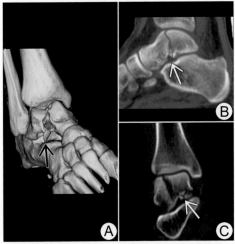

(A) 3-D rendering, (B) sagittal, and (C) coronal views of a complex talar fracture. A vertical fracture splits the talar body and dome while an oblique fracture divides the talar dome from neck. A small free fragment is seen in the sinus tarsi (arrows). Fractures cross the subtalar joint, but not the talonavicular articulation.

- Type III – Displaced neck fracture and dislocated of talar body from both subtalar and tibiotalar joints
- Osteonecrosis about 90%
- Stress fractures
  - Tarsus is 2nd most common site for stress fracture behind tibia
  - Vertical band in posterior tubercle of calcaneus, parallel to the posterior tubercle surface (i.e. attachment of Achilles tendon).
  - Talar neck
  - Best seen in reactive repair phase - ~7-10 days after injury
- Osteochondral fractures of the talar dome
  - Seen in inversion injuries of the ankle
  - Longitudinal subchondral compression fracture in the lateral talar dome oriented in the sagittal plane

Imaging Findings
General Features
- Best imaging clue: Flattening of the calcaneus on lateral view with Boehler's angle < 28°
- Linear fracture lucency across talar neck
CT Findings
- C T
  - Planar reformations for complete evaluation of fracture extent
  - Calcaneus and talus have complex geometry
    - Note displaced fragments and articulating surfaces
  - Calcaneus
    - Tongue type
    - Fracture from inferior margin of posterior facet to inferior surface
    - Horizontal fracture through posterior tubercle

- Vertical split of the posterior facet
- Centrolateral depression type
- Fracture at inferior margin of posterior facet as in tongue type
- Variable vertical or oblique fracture from inferior margin of posterior facet frees posterior facet as a separate fragment
  o Talus
    - Most fractures variably cross the neck
    - Fractures may extend to talofibular, subtalar, or talonavicular joints

MR Findings
- T2WI and proton density imaging useful for defining tendon course.
  o Tendons and ligaments hypointense on both sequences
- Fat suppressed T2 or STIR sequence may help reveal hyperintense signal of tear or partial tear

Other Modality Findings
- Nuclear medicine bone scan demonstrates increased uptake at site of occult stress fracture

Imaging Recommendations
- AP and lateral plain films identify fractures
- CT with coronal, sagittal and 3-D reformation is preferred for detailing the intricate nature of tarsal fractures, especially of the calcaneus
- MRI provides detail of tendon and ligament displacement and injury
- In cases of persistent pain and negative plain films, bone scan or MRI for evaluation of stress fracture

Differential Diagnosis
Subtalar Dislocation
- May be isolated but can coexist with talar or calcaneal fractures

Pathology
- None relevant to this case

Clinical Issues
Treatment
- Calcaneus
  o Goal is to re-establish original structure and articular geometry
  o Extra-articular fractures usually amenable to closed reduction
  o Highly comminuted fractures may not allow complete anatomic reduction. If too comminuted, closed reduction may suffice
  o If fragments lend to precise alignment, open reduction with screw and plate fixation is recommended
- Talus
  o Goal is to restore structure and restore normal articulation

Selected References
1. Barei DP et al: Fractures of the calcaneus. Orthop Clin North Am. 33(1): 263-85, 2002
2. Fortin PT et al: Talus fractures: evaluation and treatment. J Am Acad Orthop Surg. 9(2): 114-27. Review, 2001
3. Pinney SJ et al: Fractures of the tarsal bones. Orthop Clin North Am. 32(1): 21-33, 2001

Metatarsal Fractures

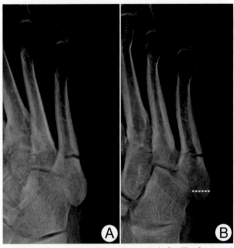

Jones fracture crosses the proximal 5th metatarsal shaft. The fracture is recognized on AP view (A), but is better seen with the metatarsals placed in the inverted oblique position (B). The avulsion fracture commonly seen in "twisted ankle" occurs more proximally at the tubercle of the metatarsal base (dashed line).

Key Facts

- Metatarsal neck and shaft fracture
  - Often direct impact mechanism by heavy object falling on foot
    - Might result from direct axial load (e.g. stubbed toe)
  - Usually transverse, oblique or comminuted - rarely longitudinal
  - Stress (march) fractures may only be evident with healing
    - Metatarsals account for ~10% of all stress fractures
    - Commonly 2nd or 3rd metatarsal neck
- Base of 5th metatarsal fractures (two types)
  - Both fractures are parallel to the short axis (transverse)
    - In children, If fracture line is parallel to the long axis on lateral base of 5th metatarsal = normal apophysis
  - Both are avulsions resulting from inversion of the foot
  - Jones fracture (Dancers fracture)
    - Lucency across the metatarsal shaft 1.5-2 cm distal to tip of the tuberosity at base of the 5th metatarsal
    - Results from plantar flexion with inversion
    - Avulsion injury from tension in lateral cord of plantar aponeurosis (connects inferolateral margin of the calcaneal tuberosity to tuberosity of 5th metatarsal)
  - Avulsion fracture
    - Peroneus brevis tendon attaches at tip of 5th metatarsal tuberosity
    - Tuberosity experiences tension at the tendon attachment on inversion of the foot
    - Tip of the tuberosity avulsed from the metatarsal base
- Lisfranc injury (Tarsometatarsal fracture dislocation)
  - Dislocation of the tarsometatarsal (Lisfranc) joint
  - Sometimes subtle – may be seen on only one view
    - Estimated that up to 20% may be missed

Metatarsal Fractures

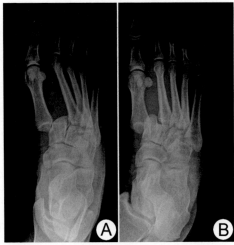

Divergent Lisfranc injury: Dislocation of the 2nd - 5th metatarsals to same side, with displacement of the 1st metatarsal to the opposite side. Metatarsals may be dorsally dislocated. AP view (A) shows dislocated 1st metatarsal, while oblique (B) shows metatarsals 2-5. Plantar load injury (e.g. fall from height, step off curb).

- Normally, metatarsal heads and calcaneal tuberosity in contact with floor with intact elevated plantar arch
- Load displaced by depression of arch, pushing the metatarsal heads and calcaneal tuberosity further apart, and forcing the hindfoot down with dorsal shear and rotation across Lisfranc joint
- Another mechanism suggests rotation of ankle and hindfoot against fixed metatarsal phalangeal complex
- Tarsometatarsal ligaments disrupted with rotation and dorsal dislocation of metatarsals
o Base of 2nd metatarsal is fractured in nearly all cases
o Commonly also a variety of compression or chip fractures of metatarsal bases and adjacent tarsal bones
o Two basic fracture configurations
  - Homolateral
  - Dislocation of 4 or all 5 metatarsals
  - Most commonly 2nd-5th
  - Rarely may be only 2 or 3 metatarsals
  - 2nd metatarsal almost always involved
  - Commonly dislocated dorsolaterally
  - Divergent dislocation
  - Dorsolateral dislocation of 2nd-5th metatarsals with medial dislocation of 1st metatarsal
  - Rarely may show medial dislocation of medial cuneiform with 1st metatarsal, with or without navicular fracture

Metatarsal Fractures

Imaging Findings

General Features
- Best imaging clue: Oblique view most helpful identifying metatarsal injury
  - View of Lisfranc joint, metatarsals and tarsus optimized
    - View of base of 5th metatarsal unobscured
    - Alignment of tarsus with individual metatarsals clear
  - Asymmetric widening or misalignment of tarsus and metatarsal
  - Fracture lucency across base of 5th metatarsal in avulsion

CT Findings
- NECT with coronal, sagittal and 3D reformations for definition of dislocated elements and identification of fine fracture fragments

MR Findings
- Helpful if concern for muscle, tendon, ligament, nerve or vessel injury
- Fat suppressed T2W or STIR images show hyperintense marrow space, ligament, tendon and muscle signal indicating edema and/or hemorrhage
- Proton density images may be helpful in identifying and following ligaments and tendons in Lisfranc injury

Other Modality Findings
- Nuclear medicine bone scan may be helpful in identifying stress fractures

Imaging Recommendations
- Plain films considered first line of evaluation
  - Should minimally include AP, lateral and oblique views
- CT prior to surgery if complex joint derangement or further clarity required in identifying fractures
- MRI to evaluate tendons and ligaments, or to assess soft tissue, vessel or nerve injury

Differential Diagnosis
Diabetic Neurotrophic Osteopathy
Charcot Osteopathy

Pathology
- None relevant to this case

Clinical Issues

Treatment
- Dislocation irreducible if entrapment of anterior tibial or peroneal tendons
- Open reduction with pin and screw fixation is preferred in Lisfranc injury
- 5th metatarsal avulsion fractures have high incidence of delayed/nonunion
  - Better result with surgical reduction and fixation

Selected References
1. Armagan OE, et al: Injuries to the toes and metatarsals. Orthop Clin North Am. 32(1): 1-10, 2001
2. Nunley JA: Fractures of the base of the fifth metatarsal: the Jones fracture. Orthop Clin North Am. 32(1): 171-80, 2001
3. Vuori JP, et al: Lisfranc joint injuries: trauma mechanisms and associated injuries. J Trauma. 35(1): 40-5, 1993

Index of Diagnoses

NOTES

NOTES

NOTES

NOTES

NOTES

NOTES

NOTES

NOTES

NOTES

NOTES

NOTES

NOTES

NOTES

NOTES

NOTES

NOTES